Joint Commission
RESOURCES

PATIENTS as PARTNERS

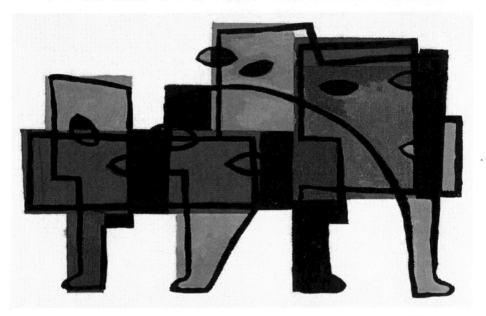

How to Involve Patients and Families in Their Own Care

Improving Health Care Quality and Safety

Editor: Meghan McGreevey
Project Manager: Andrew Bernotas
Manager, Publications: Eileen Norris
Production Manager: Johanna Harris
Associate Director: Cecily Pew
Executive Director: Catherine Chopp Hinckley
Joint Commission/JCR Reviewers: Patricia Adamski, Peter Angood, Richard Croteau, and Paul Schyve

Joint Commission Resources Mission
The mission of Joint Commission Resources is to continuously improve the safety and quality of care in the United States and in the international community through the provision of education and consultation services and international accreditation.

Joint Commission Resources educational programs and publications support, but are separate from, the accreditation activities of the Joint Commission. Attendees at Joint Commission Resources educational programs and purchasers of Joint Commission Resources publications receive no special consideration or treatment in, or confidential information about, the accreditation process.

The inclusion of an organization name, product, or service in a Joint Commission publication should not be construed as an endorsement of such organization, product, or services, nor is failure to include an organization name, product, or service to be construed as disapproval.

This publication is designed to provide accurate and authoritative information in regard to the subject matter covered. Every attempt has been made to ensure accuracy at the time of publication, however, please note that laws, regulations and standards are subject to change. Please also note that some of the examples in this publication are specific to the laws and regulations of the locality of the facility. The information and examples in this publication are provided with the understanding that the publisher is not engaged in providing medical, legal or other professional advice. If any such assistance is desired, the services of a competent professional person should be sought.

Printed in the U.S.A. 5 4 3 2 1

Requests for permission to make copies of any part of this work should be mailed to the following:
Permissions Editor
Department of Publications
Joint Commission Resources
One Renaissance Boulevard
Oakbrook Terrace, Illinois 60181
permissions@jcrinc.com

ISBN: 0-86688-996-5
Library of Congress Control Number: 2005938595

For more information about Joint Commission Resources, please visit http://www.jcrinc.com.

CONTENTS

FOREWORD

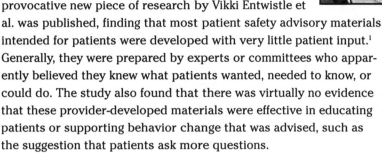

As *Patients as Partners: How to Involve Patients and Families in Their Own Care* was being developed, a provocative new piece of research by Vikki Entwistle et al. was published, finding that most patient safety advisory materials intended for patients were developed with very little patient input.[1] Generally, they were prepared by experts or committees who apparently believed they knew what patients wanted, needed to know, or could do. The study also found that there was virtually no evidence that these provider-developed materials were effective in educating patients or supporting behavior change that was advised, such as the suggestion that patients ask more questions.

Entwistle's study begs an important question underlying the entire field of patient-centered care: *Why* do we fail to include patients and their families in our safety and quality work, especially when it appears self-evident that their cooperation in following directions and participating in day-to-day care tasks is so crucial to producing good outcomes?

Most often the default answer to that question is fear of liability. But if we are honest with ourselves, that cannot be a complete response. If it were, we would be actively working with patients and families, after their liability claims were resolved, to determine what it was they experienced and what feedback they have for us. Study after study documents that patients and their families have a high desire to see their adverse experience used to prevent future harm,[2] yet we don't ask—even when it is legally safe to do so.

A deeper part of the answer is that talking with patients about safety and risk is hard and very uncomfortable work for which we lack training, skills, and tools. I will never forget my first real experience with feedback from patients and family members who had experienced medical error. I can still evoke a stomach-turning feeling as I recall it: the grief, the anger, the accusations, and—most troubling—the comparison between the victims of medical error and of the Holocaust, all surging out in a shabby conference room of a suburban Chicago hotel.

It was 1999, I was the executive director of the National Patient Safety Foundation (NPSF) at the American Medical Association, and we were the target of a rally organized by Persons United Limiting Substandards and Errors (PULSE) on behalf of victims of medical error who had been left out of the NPSF's formation two years earlier. Well acquainted with organized medicine's defensive posture vis-à-vis criticism from victims' rights advocates, I was now at the sharp end of health care providers' worst nightmare. Being likened to Nazis is a hard pill for anyone to swallow and makes for a challenging conversation-starter.

"It's a simple truth that patients and their lay caregivers see things their health care providers do not."

I had been coached well for this meeting by Doni Haas, an NPSF board member and risk manager who had shepherded a powerfully healing disclosure process in her own hospital after the death of a young boy named Ben Kolb. "What will we say to these people?" I asked her. "You don't need to worry about that," she advised, "our job is to listen."

And so we did, Haas and I, sitting in the front row for two long days as more than 100 people stepped to the podium to tell story after story of injury and disrespect. And while I felt absolutely horrible most of that time, I also recognized that our presence was enormously appreciated. We were profusely thanked for coming; a few people even expressed sympathy *for us* for how hard it must be to hear what they said. But, most important, when I was able to listen through the pain and blame, these grief-stricken people communicated in some detail a few very valuable lessons. Haas was right; our job—at least one profoundly important dimension of it—really is to listen. When we do, we learn.

It's a simple truth that patients and their lay caregivers see things their health care providers do not. True also is the fact that it is usually painful to hear from consumers who have experienced a medical error, and some of the things they say are unfair. But when we reject their communication overtures—many of which might first manifest as complaints—or funnel them into the selective fact-finding of the litigation process, we lose the treasure of their lessons learned. We also lose an often short-lived chance to regain some trust and facilitate healing for everyone involved.

I recently had the opportunity to participate in a meeting that was scheduled—as part of the settlement of a malpractice claim—between the wife of a patient who had died as the result of medical error, the CEO and risk manager of the hospital where the injury occurred, and the patient's surgeon, in whose care domain the error was made. This was a meeting that had been requested by the patient's family shortly after the adverse event, before the patient died, because the family wanted to avoid litigation. That request had been denied, either because the request was not trusted to be sincere or because the hospital insurer and the surgeon's insurer were at odds with each other about who was at fault.

On the morning the meeting was to occur, the surgeon's wife called the hospital CEO and explained that her husband could not attend. He was in their bedroom sobbing and much too distraught to face his patient's widow. Proceeding without the surgeon, the hospital CEO quoted extensively from the organization's mission statement, which emphasized patient-centered care, as well as its disclosure policy, which was intended to embody compassion. However, no apology was offered and the CEO's behavior was guarded throughout. The CEO did say the organization had taken steps to prevent a similar occurrence, but he was reluctant to discuss the details of those steps. After the meeting I debriefed with the hospital's risk manager. Both of us agreed that this event had been a missed opportunity for both learning and healing, occasioned at least in part by advice from hospital legal counsel that no apology should be made by the hospital because the adverse event was the surgeon's fault.

I share this story not to criticize either CEO or surgeon, but to underscore how daunting and irrationally fear-laden these communication episodes can be. Because the settlement papers had been signed months before, there really was no liability exposure remaining to chill the kind of person-to-person interaction that could benefit all concerned. It was fear and discomfort that prevented a conversation that was truly possible in this instance—one where compassion could naturally be expressed, accountability acknowledged, learning discussed, apologies offered, and forgiveness received.

Just as systems-based thinking is now being applied to the work of delivering care, we need to grow a better understanding of its uses in encouraging and supporting difficult communication. Even the accomplished clinician and health organization executive in this case—the latter guided by a clear mission statement and thoughtful disclosure policy—lacked the skills they needed to do this kind of thing well. Organizational support and effective tools are needed to teach, assist, and encourage.

Patients as Partners: How to Involve Patients and Families in Their Own Care is such a tool. Building on the advice of experts and the experience of health care organizations that have paved new pathways for communicating with consumers about risk in health care, it can be very useful to leaders and teachers who are committed to actualizing their patient-centered care mission statements. This book goes well beyond provider–patient interaction after an error has happened. *Patients as Partners: How to Involve Patients and Families in Their Own Care* reveals new avenues for consumer input and feedback, creating rich new potential for better prospective care as well.

In so doing, it catches a wave. There is now emerging a new appreciation for varied roles consumers can play in improving the safety and quality of care. When patients and families are included in gatherings of patient safety stakeholders, their primary contribution so far has been to share stories of harm and its impact on their lives. In the patient safety movement we have found in such stories a powerful motivational force for health care providers to focus on preventing harm as a renewed priority. However, patients have much more to offer to safety work than emotional reminders to clinicians, health care administrators, and policymakers that they too often are victims of tragic medical errors. As the new World Health Organization (WHO) Patients for Patient Safety program recognizes:

> *Important as that perspective is, a victim orientation does not position us well as partners working with health care providers to prevent harm. Indeed, the perception that patients and their families are helpless or antagonistic victims has served to distance us from playing meaningful roles in the development and*

"This book

reveals

new avenues

for consumer

input

and feedback,

creating

rich new

potential

for better

prospective

care as well."

implementation of patient safety work in the past and generated fear among some clinicians who would have otherwise engaged with us.[3]

If we agree that patients and families see aspects of system failure or vulnerability that health care workers do not, it follows that we should develop the systems-based capacity to embrace them as full partners in our safety and quality improvement work, a point of view that *Patients as Partners: How to Involve Patients and Families in Their Own Care* champions. We should include them in the development of patient education materials, our clinical training, our policy-making and facilities design, and other frontiers now being explored by the innovators profiled in *Patients as Partners: How to Involve Patients and Families in Their Own Care.*

If the invitation to consumers is made, health care is sure to find willing respondents. Again quoting the WHO Patients for Patient Safety program:

Patients and consumers who choose to partner with health care policy makers and providers are highly knowledgeable, motivated, and eager to contribute. We approach our role with a profound sense of responsibility and desire to help create a health care system that is safe, honorable, and compassionate for patients and health care workers alike. We are here to challenge health care to be truly patient-centered—especially when it is resistant to change or slow to make safer care a priority—but most fundamentally, we are here to partner to help make care better.[3]

When caring, innovative leaders reading this book invite the participation of consumers into their safety and improvement work, I cannot promise that the process will always feel heart warming or drama free. But with confidence I will guarantee that your organization will learn things about your care delivery you cannot learn anywhere else, that you will feel proud for having the courage and commitment to do difficult, patient-centered work, and that you will earn well-deserved trust from your customers.

Engaging patients with honesty about the challenges you face and the risks you manage is a profoundly important component of the care you deliver. Moreover, it is truly existential in effect. For, by doing it, you realize your mission and become what you aspire to be: an authentically patient-centered community.

—Martin J. Hatlie, J.D., president, Partnership for Patient Safety and cofounder, Consumers Advancing Patient Safety

References

1. Entwistle V.A., Mello M.M., Brennan T.A.: Advising patients about patient safety: Current initiatives risk shifting responsibility. *Jt Comm J Qual Patient Saf* 31:483–494, Sep. 2005

2. Gallagher T.H., et al.: Patients' and physicians' attitudes regarding the disclosure of medical errors. *JAMA* 289:1001–1007, Feb. 26, 2003. Hickson G.B.: Factors that prompted families to file medical malpractice claims following perinatal injuries. *JAMA* 267:1359–1363, Mar. 11, 1992. Hingorani M., Wong T., Vafidis G.: Patients' and doctors' attitudes to amount of information given after unintended injury during treatment: Cross-sectional questionnaire survey. *BMJ* 318:640–641, Mar. 6, 1999. Vincent C.A., Young M., Phillips A.: Why do people sue doctors? A study of patients and relatives taking legal action. *Lancet* 343:1609–1613, Jun. 25, 1994.

3. World Health Organization, World Alliance for Patient Safety: *Patients for Patient Safety Statement of Case.* http://www.who.int/patientsafety/patients_for_patient/statement/en/index.html (accessed Jan. 24, 2006).

INTRODUCTION

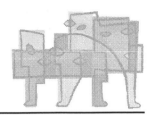

 The commitment to seeing and furthering

the innate wholeness and integrity in

every suffering human being is the true

lineage of medicine.

Rachel Naomi Remen, M.D.,
KITCHEN TABLE WISDOM

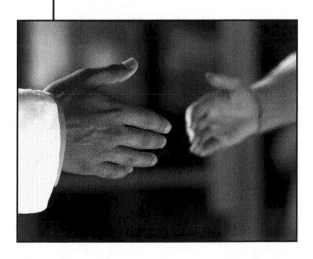

Conveying interest in and communicating with patients as individual human beings—complete with their unique histories, abilities, skills, preferences, and perspectives—is essential for developing bonds of trust between clinicians and patients; for making patients comfortable enough to share information openly and completely; for helping patients to understand, agree to, and cooperate in their treatment; and for empowering them to speak up about potential or real medical errors and hazardous conditions—in short, for improving patient safety.

Research into the most effective *ways* to involve patients in their care—that is, efforts that will lead to the best patient outcomes—is in its relative infancy.[1] Organizations such as the Agency for Healthcare Research and Quality, the Institute for Healthcare Improvement (IHI), the Robert Wood Johnson Foundation, the National Quality Forum, and the Commonwealth Fund are supporting and conducting research that will provide further evidence of the effectiveness of patient involvement.

Involving patients in their care is becoming less discretionary and more compulsory for the providers of services.[1] According to James Conway, senior fellow at the IHI and senior consultant to the Dana-Farber Cancer Institute, "There's pressure from above and pressure from below. If physicians don't get on board this train, they're going to get run over."

What is clear from experts and research conducted to date is that the commitment to improving patients' ability to understand, communicate, and act on their own behalf must start at the top of every medical organization: The leadership needs to champion open and respectful communication between clinicians and patients, and among all the staff members as well. Leaders and the staff need to create a culture of safety in which open communication can flourish and patient safety can be enhanced. The case studies and patient perspectives presented in this book illustrate the positive outcomes associated with treating patients with respect, dignity, equality, and appreciation.[2-4]

"There's pressure from above and pressure from below. If physicians don't get on board this train, they're going to get run over."

SIDEBAR

Organization Support for Patient Involvement

Pressure to improve communication and involve patients as partners in their care right now is coming from medical organizations, the federal government, and patient advocacy groups alike. The list is long and includes, among others, the following:

- Agency for Healthcare Research and Quality
- American Academy of Family Physicians
- American Medical Association
- Centers for Medicare & Medicaid Services
- Consumers Advancing Patient Safety
- CRG Medical Foundation for Patient Safety
- Institute for Family-Centered Care
- Institute for Healthcare Improvement (IHI)
- Institute of Medicine
- Joint Commission on Accreditation of Healthcare Organizations
- Medically Induced Trauma Support Services
- National Council on Patient Information and Education
- National Family Caregivers Association
- National Patient Safety Foundation (NPSF)
- National Quality Forum (NQF)
- Partnership for Patient Safety (P4PS)
- Persons United Limiting Substandards and Errors (PULSE)
- Robert Wood Johnson Foundation
- Risk Management and Patient Safety Institute
- Voice for Patients ■

Involving patients as partners in their care is more likely to be effective if the challenge is approached simultaneously on multiple fronts. Each of the following chapters focuses on a different, yet related, aspect:

- Chapter 1 explains what is meant by a culture of safety, why such a culture is the essential underpinning of patient safety, and how some organizations have succeeded in creating their own.
- Chapter 2 focuses on techniques clinicians can use to put patients at ease, initiate conversations, communicate with patients and their representatives, and gauge patient understanding.
- Chapter 3 highlights public education efforts to increase public awareness of medical errors and empower individual patient efforts to prevent them.
- Chapter 4 defines the crucial role of patients' literacy—and health literacy—in understanding their health care options and providing truly informed consent. This chapter also offers suggestions for steps medical organizations and clinicians

can take to improve patient understanding, regardless of an individual's literacy skills.

- Chapter 5 addresses the special communication needs posed by children, the elderly, and patients with chronic conditions.
- The Appendix provides a list of resources for medical organizations, clinicians, patients, and their families. These resources give further, practical information for pursuing the suggestions presented in this book.

Acknowledgments

Joint Commission Resources gratefully acknowledges the time and insights of the following people:

- Mary Ann Abrams, M.D., M.P.H., of the Health Literacy Collaborative, Iowa Health System
- Geri Amori, Ph.D., CPHRM, ARM, director of the Professional Development and Education Center at the Risk Management and Patient Safety Institute
- Margo Caulfield, codirector of the Chronic Conditions Information Network
- James Conway, senior fellow at the IHI and senior consultant to the Dana-Farber Cancer Institute
- Toni Cordell, literacy advocate
- Ilene Corina, copresident of PULSE
- Barbara Earles, R.N., M.S., CPHQ, CPHRM, director of Risk Management, Iowa Health System
- Mary Dana Gershanoff, patient literacy advocate, Boston
- Martin J. Hatlie, J.D., president of P4PS and cofounder of Consumers Advancing Patient Safety
- Matthew Mireles, Ph.D., president and director of Research at the CRG Medical Foundation for Patient Safety
- Diane Pinakiewicz, M.B.A., president of the NPSF
- Laurel Simmons, deputy director of Quality Allies at the IHI
- Elizabeth Smith, Ph.D., executive director, CRG Medical Foundation for Patient Safety
- Helen Wu, M.Sc., program director at the NQF

Special thanks to the medical writer, Eve Shapiro, for her commitment and diligence in writing this book.

References

1. Crawford M.J., et al.: Systematic review of involving patients in the planning and development of health care. *BMJ* 325:1263–1268, Nov. 30, 2002.

2. Epstein R.M., Alper B.S., Quill T.E.: Communicating evidence for participatory decision making. *JAMA* 291:2359–2366, May 19, 2004.

3. Cleaveland C.: *Sacred Space: Stories from a Life in Medicine.* Philadelphia: American College of Physicians, 1998.

4. Remen R.N.: *Kitchen Table Wisdom: Stories That Heal.* New York: Riverhead Books, 1996.

CHAPTER ONE
Including Your Patients
in a Culture of Safety

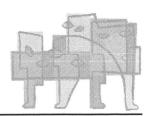

 Years ago, I took full credit when

people became well; their recovery was

testimony to my skill and knowledge as

a physician…all the time I thought

I was repairing, I was collaborating.

Rachel Naomi Remen, M.D.,
KITCHEN TABLE WISDOM

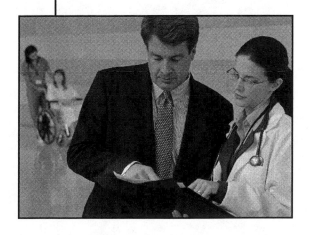

When patients and families are treated as respected partners in their health care—when patients feel free to ask questions until they understand the answers, when they feel empowered to challenge a physician or nurse about any aspect of their treatment, and when they feel supported not only by clinicians but by the entire health care organization—they are more likely to comply with treatment and have better health outcomes.[1-3] In addition, patients who are involved as partners in their care have been shown to develop better relationships with those who treat them,[4,5] are less likely to sue their physicians if things go wrong,[6] and are in a position to help prevent errors from occurring in the first place.[3,7]

Given the preponderance of evidence in its favor, why is ubiquitous patient and family involvement—known by the terms *patient-centered care, patient- and family-centered care,* or *person-centered care*—not pervasive in the United States today? Patients are demanding it and many organizations are calling for it, including the Joint

Joint Commission Requirements for Patient Involvement

National Patient Safety Goal 13
National Patient Safety Goal 13 requires disease-specific care, laboratories, and home care organizations to encourage the active involvement of patients and their families in the patient's own care as a patient safety strategy. Particularly, these organizations need to define and communicate the means for patients and their families to report concerns about safety and encourage them to do so (Requirement 13A). Although the Joint Commission made this goal applicable to a few select types of organizations, patient involvement is certainly relevant to all care settings.*

Interactive communication with patients and families about all aspects of their care, treatment, or services is an important characteristic in a culture of safety. When patients are engaged as active participants in their own care, they are more aware of possible complications and treatment choices. Patients and their families can be an important source of feedback about actual or potential adverse events because, with their unique perspective, they often observe things that busy health care providers may not. By encouraging communication about errors or

* The applicability of this goal is subject to change based on annual revisions to the National Patient Safety Goals. Please see *Joint Commission Perspectives* for the most up-to-date information on the National Patient Safety Goals.

near misses, patients and their families can be effectively integrated into an organization's patient safety work processes.

Compliance Solutions for Implementing Goal 13

Just as organizational cultures are changing to promote a safer environment, patients are also changing to become more active in their own care. When educated properly, patients and families seem to welcome the opportunity to contribute to improve communication and prevent breakdowns in the system. For example, patients and families can play important roles in helping their health care providers (1) reach an accurate diagnosis, (2) ensure that treatment plans are appropriate and effective, and (3) identify side effects or adverse events quickly and take appropriate action. Organization reporting systems that do not provide pathways for patient reporting miss the opportunity to capture information that can contribute to error-prevention and quality-improvement work.

The following tips can help improve patient communication and education:

• Tell patients and their families that the single most important way they can help health care providers to prevent errors is to be active members of the health care team. Tell them how they can participate and encourage them to do so.

Continued on page 10

Commission, particularly through its National Patient Safety Goal 13 (*see* Sidebar 1.1 on pages 8–12 for more information about Goal 13).

The purpose of this chapter is to explain how health care organizations and clinicians can include patients and families as partners in their health care. Health care organizations are moving from a traditional model of health care delivery, in which the staff works independently, to a model that thoroughly integrates patients and their families into the health care team. But this shift is a process that requires discussion and planning, which typically cannot be accomplished overnight. Change requires an honest assessment of the way things are currently done in an organization, a vision of the way things could be done, the setting of practical and achievable goals, and thoughtful planning to move the proposed changes forward. Sweeping changes in an organization's culture may be required to transform it from a traditional model of care into one that is truly patient-centered—in other words, into a culture of safety.

Planning

and action at

every level

of the

organization,

from the

top down,

will be

needed to

create a

culture of

safety.

Creating a Culture of Safety

A culture of safety is one in which preventing harm to patients is paramount. Creating a culture of safety involves breaking down barriers and leveling an often uneven playing field so that executives, administrators, clinicians, and patients and their families treat each other as partners on one team—a team that has mutual respect for and trust in one another—with the goal of ensuring patient safety and satisfaction.

The concept is simple, but its implementation may not be. In organizations in which the focus has been on the needs of health care professionals, putting the focus back on patients may take some organizational reevaluation and restructuring on the part of executives, administrators, and boards, and some self-reflection on the part of physicians, nurses, and everyone responsible for patient care.[2] Changes in philosophy, attitude, and behavior may be required. Planning and action at every level of the organization, from the top down, will be needed to create a culture of safety.[8]

SIDEBAR 1.1

Joint Commission Requirements for Patient Involvement, continued

- Provide explicit, clear information to patients and their families about the risks associated with their particular procedures or courses of care, and what to watch out for during or after particular conditions, procedures, or courses of care. This information should be presented both orally and in writing. Just as important as providing this information is ensuring that patients and their family members understand it.

- Provide clear, easy-to-understand written information about the side effects that a medicine could cause; this will better prepare patients if known side effects do occur or if something unexpected happens. Encourage patients to report a problem right away so they can get help before the problem gets worse.

- Tell patients they should not assume that no news is good news after they have a test. Patients can help by asking about their test results and letting their providers know when they don't receive them when promised.

- Encourage patients and their families to speak up about any concerns they have about errors, potential errors, or the quality of their care.

- Encourage patients and their families to learn about their conditions and treatments by asking their physicians and nurses, and by using other reliable sources recommended by their health care providers.

Standards Relating to Patient Involvement

Please also note that there are other Joint Commission requirements relevant to patient involvement, including the following:

Accreditation Participation Requirement 8

The organization provides notices to its public that when an individual has any concerns about patient care and safety in the organization, that the organization has not addressed, he or she is encouraged to contact the organization's management.

RI.2.30 Patients are involved in decisions about care, treatment, and services provided.

RI.2.40 Informed consent is obtained.

RI.2.90 Patients and, when appropriate, their families are informed about the outcomes of care, treatment, and services that have been provided, including unanticipated outcomes.

PC.6.10 The patient receives education and training specific to the patient's needs and as appropriate to the care, treatment, and services provided.

Continued on page 12

Experts agree that creating a culture of safety must start with executive leadership and be evident in every interaction between clinicians and patients and in every interaction among clinicians themselves.[8] Creating a culture of safety involves imposing personal and organizational accountability but not blame, publicly acknowledging errors either made or narrowly missed, and seeing them as opportunities to learn and to improve. According to Diane Pinakiewicz, M.B.A., president of the National Patient Safety Foundation, "Fostering a culture of safety needs to involve visionary as well as practical leadership."

When one enters into a culture of safety, according to patient literacy advocate, Mary Dana Gershanoff, you know it right away: Signs are posted in every room telling patients it's all right to ask your physician or nurse if they've washed their hands—and clinicians welcome and encourage such questions. Patients feel comfortable asking the person who will wheel them into the operating suite to first check their identification bracelets to be sure they have the right patient—and the person who is asked does so. Patients and their families are treated with the dignity and respect that characterize interactions among everyone in such an organization. Patients and family members are

> **Tip** Post signs in the hallways and rooms that patients use to encourage their family members to ask questions or voice concerns about their safety.

encouraged to report safety concerns and, according to Martin J. Hatlie, J.D., president of the Partnership for Patient Safety and cofounder of Consumers Advancing Patient Safety, "Clinicians are taught to listen past any anger or frustration for the safety content of the message."

In organizations that have established cultures of safety, patient and family involvement has resulted in the commissioning of new services, including advocacy and crisis services. Such results have, in turn, positively influenced staff attitudes toward involving patients and families as partners in their care, further deepening the culture of safety in these organizations.

> **Tip** Communication changes have worked to improve safety in the aviation industry. According to Diane Pinakiewicz, M.B.A., president of the National Patient Safety Foundation, "The health care industry has learned a lot from the aviation industry in moving the safety ball forward."

Change, even necessary change, can be uncomfortable for organizations and individuals. But what is the alternative? In light of the evidence[6] that a culture of blame, acrimony, and generally strained relations among staff members—and failure to communicate openly and respectfully with patients—contributes to medical errors, change is an essential first step in prevention.

Creating a Community of Competence

A community of competence—a multidisciplinary, cross-functional, and cohesive community—is one in which the risk of harm may be anticipated and managed by bringing together highly skilled, knowledgeable, and experienced professionals who, with respect for one another, view problems and seek solutions from different perspectives. A community of competence is essential for a culture of safety to flourish.

"A first step in creating a community of competence," says Elizabeth Smith, Ph.D., executive director of the CRG Medical Foundation for Patient Safety, "is to understand the unique needs and concerns of patients and their families. Only then can health care professionals work together in patient-centered teams to provide the safe, high-quality, timely, and equitable care that patients deserve and pay for." Smith also stresses the importance of the organization's chief executive officer and executive team to be "champions for change—to create, accept, and openly support the movement toward a just culture."

The Costs of Not Creating a Culture of Safety

According to Hatlie, the highest cost of not creating a culture of safety is "poor outcomes—patient deaths or injuries that could have been avoided." "Whether patients admitted to the emergency department live or die"[6] or, as Hatlie adds, "enjoy future quality of life or struggle with disability," is directly related to the quality of the communications and interactions among the emergency department staff. In organizations in which health care professionals have mutual respect for each other's skills and communicate openly with one another, patients are released earlier than they are in organizations in which clinicians are less trusting, less communicative, and less respectful.[6]

Another cost of not creating a culture of safety, Pinakiewicz notes, is the reinforcement of the public's mistrust of clinicians, the health care industry, and the care delivered: "The public's

> *"Clinicians are taught to listen past any anger or frustration for the safety content of the message."*

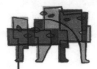

image comes from the news media. Patients hear bad stories in the news, are afraid, and then see providers as the enemy." There is a common public perception that health care professionals are unresponsive to patients' questions and concerns.[9] To empower patients to participate actively in their own care, many government agencies, private organizations, and associations encourage patients and their families to ask their physicians questions, especially when they are concerned that an error is about to be (or may have been) made.

When asked, appropriate responses are required from clinicians if questions are to be effective in helping to prevent errors. Physicians and nurses need to be willing not only to answer questions, but also must be willing to check their actions in responding. Patients have been harmed by health care professionals who have ignored rather than responded to a patient's or family's concerns.[9]

Patients who have been ignored, rather than responded to, do not feel like partners in their care. According to an unnamed safety improvement specialist, "Systems aren't set up to have you involved. You have to bully your way in to be a partner. And you're really not a partner; you're an imposition at that point. And patients feel that."[9] And, according to some researchers, "Patient involvement does not appear among the main types of actions that hospital executives are implementing to improve patient safety. Beyond distributing advice for patients ["usually," Hatlie adds, "prepared without much patient input"], little has been done to support systems change or encourage health care professionals to facilitate greater or more effective involvement of patients in their own care—for the sake of safety or otherwise."[9]

> **Tip** Many organizations have developed fact sheets that include advice and questions designed to foster patient and family participation in their care, including the following:
>
> - Agency for Healthcare Research and Quality (http://www.ahrq.gov)
> - American Academy of Family Physicians (http://www.aafp.org)
> - American College of Physicians (http://www.acponline.org)
> - Chronic Conditions Information Network of Vermont and New Hampshire (http://www.cc-info.net)
> - Joint Commission on Accreditation of Healthcare Organizations (http://www.jcaho.org)
> - Massachusetts Coalition for the Prevention of Medical Errors (http://www.macoalition.org)
> - National Family Caregivers Association (http://www.nfcacares.org)
>
> *See* the Appendix for Web sites of these and other organizations, which includes links to sample fact sheets and other resources for patients, clinicians, and medical institutions.

The reticence many patients feel about asking questions—often life-saving questions—which they think may be viewed by a physician or nurse as challenging, cannot be underestimated. Patients may be afraid of being treated dismissively, or afraid that their physician may not want to treat them if they are perceived as being "difficult." They may be so intimidated by the attitudes and behaviors of those who treat them that they subsume their concerns about their own health to their concerns about the needs of their physicians. The results can be failure on the part of patients to respond quickly on their own behalf.[10] According to James Conway, senior fellow at the Institute for Healthcare Improvement and senior consultant to the Dana-Farber Cancer Institute, there is increasing pressure from consumer groups to put the focus where it belongs—to make patient-centered care the rule rather than the exception. He says, "Organizations and clinicians will have no choice but to change and participate in what has become a vocal and persistent patient movement." Perhaps the most effective way to respond to this movement is to create and nurture patient and family advisory councils.

Creating a Patient and Family Advisory Council

Institutions such as the Dana-Farber Cancer Institute, Brigham and Women's Hospital, and the Medical College of Georgia (MCG) view patients and their families as integral parts of their larger institutional family and demonstrate this daily by supporting and working with their patient and family advisory councils.

Sometimes, as was the case with these institutions, the impetus to begin involving patients and families in organizational decision making begins with the organization's leadership. In other cases, patients and families are the driving force. Either way, integrating patients and families as partners is a process that takes time. This process depends on creating communities of competence and on establishing relationships of open communication and mutual trust among leaders, administrators, the staff, and patients. As Patricia Reid Ponte and colleagues have noted, the ability of a health care organization to work in true partnership with patients and their families depends first on building a foundation for effective teamwork

"Systems aren't set up to have you involved. You have to bully your way in to be a partner. And you're really not a partner; you're an imposition at that point. And patients feel that."

throughout the organization itself. This foundation must be built and supported by the executive leadership and characterize every inter-action among staff and interactions between staff members and patients and their families. Only then can the enterprise of formaliz-ing relationships among administration, the staff, and patients by establishing patient and family advisory councils begin.[8]

When the time is right, it may be best to start small. Small work groups can solve specific problems informally and can naturally lead to larger, more formalized patient and family advisory councils over time (these bodies also may be called family advisory boards, family-pro-fessional councils, consumer advocacy boards, and the like). And, as Hatlie notes, "Some organi-zations have moved toward calling them partner-ship councils or boards, to underscore that their role is more than merely advisory."

Tip To start, organizations should work with patients on an applicable patient safety initiative or project. Thereafter, staff members can use those lessons learned to create a patient and family advisory council for the entire organization.

When the decision is made to create a patient and family advi-sory council, the Institute for Family-Centered Care suggests the following steps be taken:

- Talk with people who have been involved in such councils at other institutions, learn what they've done, and get sample materials they've produced.
- Convene a core planning group of families and staff members that includes people of different cultures, races, religions, ages, and educational and socioeconomic backgrounds.
- Discuss the purpose, structure, and goals of the group.
- Arrange a meeting between the organization's leadership and members of the core planning group to discuss goals, support, and logistics.
- Announce formation of the council at staff meetings, through newsletters, and on the organization's Web site.
- Encourage staff members, patients, and families to bring issues to the council.

In developing a patient and family advisory council, it is impor-tant to decide on and put in writing the group's operating principles, organizational structure, total number of members (including a diverse mix of patients, family members, and staff members), the senior leaders of the organization" to be involved, and the staff liaison to support council activities. It is helpful to invite a variety of staff members to attend meetings to give their perspectives on specific topics. Other important issues that need to be resolved and put in writing include terms of council membership, attendance requirements, responsibilities of members, and compensation and reimbursement for expenses.

> **JOINT COMMISSION STANDARD**
>
> **RI.2.30** Patients are involved in decisions about care, treatment, and services provided.

General Guidelines for Council Membership: Patients and Family Members

The patient and family advisory council at Dana-Farber and Brigham and Women's Hospital looks for members who are experienced in collaborating with professionals and with members of the broader community, who are comfortable expressing their opinions in a group, and who actively and openly listen to the opinions of others. They seek members who will be enthusiastic about the cancer center and its mission, but who will also be able to view the center objectively and critically and to constructively express criticisms and suggestions. Potential members should be concerned not only with their own experiences, but concerned broadly with the experiences of other patients and families.[8]

General Guidelines for Council Membership: Staff Liaison

According to the Institute for Family-Centered Care, "Key attitudes and qualities of a staff liaison include patience, perseverance, flexibility,

> **Tip** Post signs in the hallways and rooms that patients use to encourage their family members to ask questions or voice concerns about their safety.

listening skills, openness to new ideas, a willingness to learn and to teach, the ability to work positively and proactively, the ability to see strengths in all people and situations and to build on these strengths, and a sense of humor."[11]

The Institute for Family-Centered Care provides a wealth of information and materials, in print and on its Web site, to help those who are interested in developing and sustaining patient and family advisory councils. More information is available at http://www.familycenteredcare.org.

Educating Physicians About Communicating in a Culture of Safety

How can medical organizations and practicing clinicians who want to improve their communication skills with patients and colleagues, so essential in a culture of safety, learn how to do this? One answer is through the Kenneth B. Schwartz Center Rounds—a program for health professionals designed to enhance and support improved communication and to strengthen relationships between clinicians and patients and among clinicians themselves. "All too often as providers we simply provide care and do not take time to see how it impacts our own psyche and personality," says Clifford M. Sales, M.D., M.B.A., FACS, chief of the Division of Vascular Surgery at Overlook Hospital in Summit, New Jersey. "The Rounds are a wonderful outlet that bring us back to the place where we really are in medicine but all too

SIDEBAR 1.2

The MCG Medical Center and the MCG Children's Medical Center

Through the input of pediatric nurses and committed leaders, The Medical College of Georgia (MCG) Medical Center in Augusta, Georgia, has been practicing patient- and family-centered care successfully since 1993. When an assessment revealed that providers' concerns superseded the concerns of patients and their families, the organization made a commitment to introduce family-centered care on pediatric units.

First, the leadership, administrators, and staff members educated themselves about patient- and family-centered care. Then they brought families into the process by holding a "visioning retreat," where participants came to a consensus about their philosophy, values, and priorities. Following this retreat, families were appointed to all design planning committees. A Family-Centered Services Committee that included staff members, faculty, and families was created to explore ways to integrate family-centered concepts and strategies into all aspects of the MCG's Children's Medical Center. This committee evolved into the Family Advisory Council, which continues to provide guidance for policy and program development.

In 1996 the MCG Children's Medical Center created the Children's Advisory Council, known as Kids'

SIDEBAR 1.2

ART (Architectural and Recreational Team). Past and current pediatric patients share their ideas and, in so doing, have influenced design, policy, and attitudes among the staff. Their contributions led to the selection of the Children's Medical Center logo, new hospital menus, the raising of money to purchase new toys for outpatient clinics, and articles describing their experiences as patients in several hospital publications.

Building on the success of their efforts, the MCG implemented patient- and family-centered care throughout the institution in 1997. They created an Adult Family Forum that evolved into the MCG Health Partners Advisory Council. And, in 1998, the hospital created the position of Director of Family Services Development. As part of the MCG's management team, this director ensures that patient and family perspectives are represented in all aspects of the health care experience for children and adults.

Today, patient- and family-centered care continues to thrive and expand in services that include the Augusta Multiple Sclerosis Center, the MCG Neuroscience Center of Excellence, and the Breast Health Suite. For the Breast Health Suite, a woman with breast cancer served on the planning committee to design and build a new mammography center.

Her participation and insight changed the way health care professionals viewed this center, helping to

Continued on page 20

often forget . . . people caring for people, helping another human to get better or to tolerate their life just a bit more." The Schwartz Center Rounds, which can be incorporated successfully into any medical organization that has support from its top leaders and commitment from its staff, have addressed topics such as the following:

- How to discuss a do-not-resuscitate order with a patient and family
- When cultural and religious beliefs interfere with your ability to communicate
- Breakdowns in communication between patients and caregivers
- Care of the elderly: assumptions and challenges
- Race and the patient-caregiver relationship
- Are we connecting with our patients or are we too busy?
- Delivering bad news
- How it feels when a patient "fires" you
- Medical mistakes
- Humor and healing
- Putting compassion to the test: what to do when you do not want to walk into the room

"Patients want people to be kind, to understand them and treat them as human beings. They don't want to be the 'leg' in room 10. That's one of the most important things that Rounds do. They make us all human."[12]

In a culture of safety, not only do physicians educate patients, but patients educate physicians. At Dana-Farber and Brigham and Women's Hospital, the adult patient and family advisory council has developed and implemented an educational program for first-year oncology fellows. Council members converse with the fellows about the cancer patient's experience. The group provides a forum where patients and fellows can interact and share comments, anxieties, or concerns about the relationship between physicians and their patients and families. The MCG began its Patient and Family Faculty Program in 2003. As part of this program, families share their stories with students, trainees, and staff members to teach them about the importance of patient- and family-centered care and to help them learn how to implement it.

For the next generation of clinicians to learn the importance of effectively communicating with patients, medical schools play a crucial role. But how common are communications courses in medical schools today? There are differences of opinion on this point. Matthew Mireles, Ph.D., president and director of Research, and executive director Smith of the CRG Medical Foundation for Patient Safety say such courses aren't common enough. According to Smith, teaching students how to communicate effectively with patients does not seem to be commonplace in U.S. medical schools, and the barrier is the medical school curriculum.

> ## SIDEBAR 1.2
>
> ### The MCG Medical Center and the MCG Children's Medical Center, continued
>
> make it a place for women's health and wellness, rather than simply a diagnostic and treatment center.
>
> Key to the success of patient- and family-centered care at the MCG is the organization's ongoing evaluation of patient satisfaction. Their commitment to continuous improvement has placed The MCG's Children's Medical Center consistently in the 90th percentile or higher for patient satisfaction, compared to more than 50 children's hospitals on a national measurement of patient satisfaction. ∎

"The patient is still left out because the curriculum is so rushed," Smith says. "It is hard to find the time to consider the patient. The only hope for including the perspective of the whole patient and family in medical care is to get students involved." In addition, Mireles says, "We need to expose medical students to the importance of communication. They need to understand the importance of being involved with patients' stories, to appreciate the patient as a person." Mireles suggests that teaching communication skills should start early in a medical student's career, as early as the first year.

William Jacott, M.D., special adviser for Professional Relations at the Joint Commission, who teaches a course at the University of Minnesota Medical School (Minneapolis) titled "The Physician and Society," agrees that such education is essential. But, unlike Smith and Mireles, he believes that such courses are being offered more widely in medical schools than ever before. "The course 'The Physician and Society' covers medical-ethical and medical-legal issues and communication," says Jacott. "It is now part of the curriculum in many medical schools. It has been offered for the last three years at Minnesota and students love it. It is their first taste of what it's like to be in clinical medicine. Medical students now have more role models for good communication than they have had in the past."

Jacott, Smith, and Mireles agree that the ability to communicate well with patients has practical importance, and the consequences of inadequate communication are profound. As Jacott says, "Patients want information and they want it clear. Physicians need to speak the language that the patient can understand." As Mireles cautions, "If patients don't think their physician has understood them—or if they don't understand what their physician has told them—they will look for advice and medical information elsewhere, including the Internet. These sites may not be the most accurate places to get medical information."

Clif Cleaveland, M.D., an internist practicing in Chattanooga, Tennessee, puts it this way in his book, *Sacred Space:* "Patients are not diseases but human beings with complex histories who happen

"Medical students now have more role models for good communication than they have had in the past."

to have experienced illness or injury. . . .Without this awareness, we are at risk of processing rather than treating those who seek our help."[13]

Creating a culture of safety depends on effective communication at all levels. Consider this statement: "My physician colleagues and I cherish and respect personal, ongoing, confidential dealings with our patients. Intonations of speech and facial expression tell what lies beyond our patients' descriptions of their symptoms and fears. Our styles of listening, explaining, and comforting must be carefully tailored to the complex needs of each individual patient."[13] And as Rachel Naomi Remen, M.D., says, "As physicians, we have been trained to value and develop the intellect, but the parts we have sacrificed to our expertise—the heart, the emotions, the soul and the intuition—are basic human strengths. We will need to find ways to respect and develop these strengths."

References

1. Coulter A.: After Bristol: Putting patients at the centre. *Qual Saf Health Care* 11:186–188, Jun. 2002.

2. Beach M.C., et al.: Do patients treated with dignity report higher satisfaction, adherence, and receipt of preventive care? *Ann Fam Med* 3:331–338, Jul.–Aug. 2005.

3. Anthony R., et al.: John M. Eisenberg Patient Safety Awards. The LVHHN Patient Safety Video: Patients as Partners in Safe Health Care Delivery. *Jt Comm J Qual Saf* 29:640–645, Dec. 2003.

4. Epstein R.M., Alper B.S., Quill T.E.: Communicating evidence for participatory decision making. *JAMA* 291:2359–2366, May 19, 2004.

5. Kuzel A.J., et al.: Patient reports of preventable problems and harms in primary health care. *Ann Fam Med* 2:333–340, Jul.–Aug. 2005.

6. Rubin I.: Interpersonal relationships: The "soft stuff" of patient safety. In Youngberg B.J, Hatlie M.J. (eds.): *The Patient Safety Handbook*. Sudbury, MA: Jones and Bartlett, 2004.

7. American Academy of Family Physicians: *Medical errors: Tips to help prevent them*. http://familydoctor.org/736.xml (accessed Nov. 1, 2005).

8. Ponte P.R., et al.: Making patient-centered care come alive: Achieving full integration of the patient's perspective. *J Nurs Adm* 33:82–90, Feb. 2003.

9. Entwistle V.A., Mello M.M., Brennan T.A.: Advising patients about patient safety: Current initiatives risk shifting responsibility. *Jt Comm J Qual Patient Saf* 31:483–494, Sep. 2005.

10. Hibbard J.H., et al.: Can patients be part of the solution? Views on their role in preventing medical errors. *Med Care Res Rev* 62:601–616, Oct. 2005.

11. Weber P.D., Johnson B.H.: *Developing and Sustaining a Patient and Family Advisory Council.* Bethesda, MD: Institute for Family-Centered Care, 2000.

12. Bishko A.: The emotional side of healing: The Kenneth B. Schwartz Center uses rounds to promote compassionate healthcare. *On Call* Jun. 2005.

13. Cleaveland C.: *Sacred Space: Stories from a Life in Medicine.* Philadelphia: American College of Physicians, 1998.

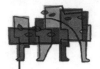
CASE STUDY 1.1
METAMORPHOSIS AT THE DANA-FARBER CANCER INSTITUTE

ARTICLE AT A GLANCE

Name of the organizations:
Dana-Farber Cancer Institute, Brigham and Women's Hospital (whose collaboration is referred to as the Dana-Farber/Brigham and Women's Cancer Center or DF/BWCC), and the Children's Hospital Boston (whose collaboration is referred to as Dana-Farber/Children's Hospital Cancer Center or DF/CHCC), three hospitals in Boston that collaborate to provide adult and pediatric cancer care.

Purpose of the project:
The organizations sought to increase patient participation in all aspects of hospital functioning and make patients and families true partners in identifying and resolving problems, thereby enhancing patient safety and satisfaction.

Lessons learned:
Active patient involvement improves the quality of care, enhances patient self-esteem, increases patient safety, and reduces the potential for medical errors.

Outcomes:
DF/BWCC's and DF/CHCC's efforts to cultivate patient involvement in all aspects of their care have resulted in the creation of increasing opportunities for patient and family involvement.

Staff involved:
Hospital leadership at the highest levels and all health care professionals.

"Nothing good happens until something bad happens," the saying goes. Nowhere did this prove to be truer than at the Dana-Farber Cancer Institute in Boston. In late November 1994, two women—Betsy Lehman, a reporter for the Boston Globe, and Maureen Bateman—received, in one day, four times the daily dose of chemotherapy for breast cancer. Betsy Lehman died on December 3 as a direct result of this massive overdose; Maureen Bateman suffered permanent heart damage and died several years later of cancer. These medical errors reverberated in investigations, suspensions, and then lawsuits. Finally, these errors became the catalyst for Dana-Farber to initiate organizationwide changes, with patients playing key roles to ensure patient safety. The changes made at Dana-Farber, from the top down, have placed them in the pantheon of patient safety.

Their Plan to Involve Patients
Administrators at Dana-Farber put their plan for patient involvement into action in 1996, with small steps in the discrete project of combining and moving cancer care services between Dana-Farber Cancer Institute and Brigham and Women's Hospital in Boston. Administrators at both hospitals invited patients and families to serve on planning committees and to oversee the creation of

CASE STUDY 1.1

what was to become the Dana-Farber/Brigham and Women's Cancer Center (DF/BWCC). Thereafter, Dana-Farber collaborated with the Children's Hospital Boston to create the Dana-Farber/Children's Hospital Cancer Center (DF/CHCC).

Despite initial staff hesitation to involve patients in the planning and moving process, staff members came to see that patients played an important role in offering suggestions and resolving problems and began to see the value of making patients partners in this enterprise. The success of this effort became the catalyst for asking for and then incorporating patient suggestions at all levels and across all domains of the organization. With their leadership teams serving as champions, the three organizations created a patient and family advisory council to ensure that patient ideas would be included in the organization's policies and procedures, daily decisions, purchases, hirings, and especially quality of care.

The patient and family advisory council mission statement has guided everything the members have done and continue to do:

"The council's mission is to assure the delivery of the highest standard of comprehensive and compassionate health care. To do so, members work in partnership with health care providers to:

- Strengthen communication and collaboration among patients, families, caregivers, and staff
- Promote patient and family advocacy and involvement
- Propose and participate in developing oncology programs, services, and policies."[1]

Creating Patient and Family Advisory Councils

Dana-Farber created two patient and family advisory councils—first with Brigham and Women's for adult care and then with Children's Hospital Boston for pediatric care. The adult and

Staff members came to see that patients played an important role in offering suggestions and resolving problems.

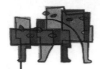

pediatric patient and family advisory councils, as well as a variety of committees on which patients and family members are invited to serve, are the mechanisms by which patients and family members work collaboratively with hospital staff and administrators to continuously improve patient care, hospital operations, staff education, staff hiring, and more. Members of the patient and family advisory councils accompany physicians on patient rounds and are welcome to ask patients about their care experience; they relate patients' comments to the hospital staff through staff liaisons who attend patient and family advisory council meetings. Staff liaisons support patient and family advisory council members as they work with administrators and staff to influence hospital policies, programs, and practices.

The patient and family advisory council members are charged with providing feedback on patient care, program planning, organizational priorities, and decision making. Through the mechanism of the patient and family advisory councils, patients and families of the DF/BWCC and DF/CHCC have a voice in determining how clinical services are structured, how ambulatory units are designed, how bills are formatted, and how buildings are maintained.

The Impact of the Advisory Councils

Patient involvement at DF/BWCC and DF/CHCC has resulted in a greater sense of equality between patients and providers at all levels, including that of direct patient care. By viewing patients and families as partners, more open patient–provider communication, earlier identification of potential problems, and development of more effective solutions to problems have been possible.

Specifically, patient and family involvement has resulted in the production of new or improved sources of patient information, simplifying of appointment procedures, extending opening

CASE STUDY 1.1

times, improving transportation to treatment units, and improving access for people with disabilities.

As one example of the achievements of the patient and family advisory councils, adult council members learned that patients with neutropenia who were admitted after office hours often experienced long waits in the emergency department. (Neutropenia is an abnormal decrease in white blood cells most often resulting from a viral infection or exposure to certain drugs or chemicals.) These waits were not only exhausting but also delayed the start of treatment. Working through the staff liaison, the patient and family advisory council formed a work team that included council members, nurses, physicians, and staff from admitting, medical records, and the emergency department. Together, the team analyzed patient satisfaction data, patient flow, and other factors associated with the admissions process. Their work resulted in recommendations for a modified process that involved using the telephone to screen patients at home and then directly admitting selected patients to the inpatient units, thus bypassing the emergency department altogether.[8]

The adult and pediatric patient and family advisory councils can also be credited with the following achievements:

- Launched the quarterly newsletter for patients, *Side by Side*
- Helped design treatment, program, and common areas
- Launched a "patients as educators" program for nurses and physicians
- Suggested ways to shorten patient waiting times
- Advocated for increased psychosocial support services
- Identified the need for greater privacy in outpatient areas
- Worked with the accounting department to create more patient-friendly billing statements

As important as these achievements are, hospital administrators say there is more to be done. As Patricia Reid Ponte and colleagues note, "A larger challenge than involving patients and

CASE STUDY 1.1

their families in health care organizations relates to how our organization can bring the concepts of collaborative, shared decision-making and partnership to the individual patient–provider relationship. To our advantage, our clinicians embrace these concepts philosophically and welcome the chance to include patients and family members in the organization's efforts to reshape aspects of day-to-day care."[2]

DF/BWCC and DF/CHCC have the support of their health care professionals for making patients and their families an integral part of the health care they provide. To achieve patient-centered care, organizations must have the enthusiastic and committed support of each and every member of the staff from the top down, and the dedicated participation of patients and their families.

References

1. Weber P.D., Johnson B.H.: *Developing and Sustaining a Patient and Family Advisory Council.* Bethesda, MD: Institute for Family-Centered Care, 2000.

2. Ponte P.R., et al.: Making patient-centered care come alive: Achieving full integration of the patient's perspective. *J Nurs Adm* 33:82–90, Feb. 2003.

PATIENT PERSPECTIVE 1.1

THE DANA-FARBER CANCER INSTITUTE'S COMMITMENT TO PATIENT-CENTERED CARE

Mary Dana Gershanoff was treated for cancer as an outpatient at the Dana-Farber Cancer Institute between 2000 and 2001. Co-chair of the institute's patient and family advisory council, she shares her perspectives on the organization's patient- and family-centered approach to health care:

"The first time I walked into the Dana-Farber Cancer Institute I was immediately aware of the difference between this hospital and everywhere else. Even the parking attendants were nice. Other patients have said this to me, too. The parking attendants are the first people you see when you go for cancer treatment and the last people you see when you leave. It may seem like a small thing, but their being nice gives you an impression about the hospital before you walk in the door and is comforting when you leave. The fact that the parking attendants are nice shows there is top-level support for kindness. When you walk into the building, if you look lost, you're apt to have a volunteer or staff person offer to help you.

I never had a physician look at his watch while I was there. The physicians concentrated on me. I would come in with a list of questions and they took all the time I needed. I felt a willingness, a responsiveness. My surgeon was amazing. He explained the treatment options, recommended a treatment plan, and then said the choice was mine. He handed me a card with his home phone number written on the back and said, "If you have any questions or want to talk about this, call me." I never did call him at home, but it made me feel better knowing that I could.

I became involved with the patient and family advisory council because I had such an excellent experience at Dana-Farber that I wanted to give back. Dana-Farber has signs in the elevators giving interested patients a phone number to call. I spoke to a council member and was interviewed by staff members and a member of the council. They want to be careful that members of the patient

"He handed me a card with his home phone number written on the back . . . I never did call him at home, but it made me feel better knowing that I could."

PATIENT PERSPECTIVE 1.1

"... a physician on the committee told me he 'was very skeptical when you first came in here. But I appreciate it now, you bring a different perspective.'"

and family advisory council work in partnership with the staff to make Dana-Farber a better place; they want to create and maintain a positive atmosphere.

The patient and family advisory council helps to improve the overall environment at Dana-Farber. There is often some hesitation by patients to speak up to their providers, so there's something to be said for patients having other patients to talk to. Because clinicians get used to their environment, they do not see things that patients would see (for example, clinicians may not notice that a door is too heavy or that the toilet seat is askew). These are not noticeable issues for the staff, but they are noticeable to patients.

The council is unique in that its members are truly embedded in the structure of Dana-Farber. There's not a committee on which patients are not represented. This shows a level of trust in the patient and family advisory council and says wonderful things about Dana-Farber. To demonstrate the top-level commitment, four Dana-Farber staff members sit on the patient and family advisory council: the Chief Medical Officer, the Chief Nurse, the person responsible for patient and family relations, and the staff liaison. When you have people as important as the Chief Medical Officer and the Chief Nurse attend your meetings, it is a sign of solid support.

Members of the patient and family advisory council are working on standardizing emergency information forms across centers, since each center uses different forms—and every patient should have the same information, such as whom to call for help in an emergency. Council members also are represented on a committee working on preventing falls from elevator doors and other causes. And we are involved in fun things like design of waiting rooms. When a carpet had been ordered that patients on the council reacted negatively to, the carpet was returned.

We are even on the Quality Improvement–Risk Management Committee, a trustee-level committee whose members discuss things that go wrong. I am now part of a team working on a document having to do with disclosure, called "When Things Go Wrong." Initially there was hesitation to involve us on this committee, which includes the staff from Dana-Farber, Beth Israel

PATIENT PERSPECTIVE 1.1

Deaconness Medical Center, and Massachusetts General Hospital. But last month, I felt we had been accepted when a physician on the committee told me he "was very skeptical when you first came in here. But I appreciate it now, you bring a different perspective." Physicians at these meetings ask the patients on the council what we'd want to hear if things go wrong. We discuss how apology should be made. The disclosure document will be circulated to hospitals in Boston—each one will have its own implementation, but they want to have a standard approach to what should be done when things go wrong."

Finally, Gershanoff notes, "We're on the leading edge of a real sea-change in the relationships between patients and physicians. This is all for the good."

CHAPTER TWO
Opening the Lines of Communication

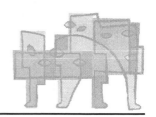

 I suspect that the most basic and powerful way to connect to another person is to listen. Just listen. . . . When people are talking, there's no need to do anything but receive them.

Rachel Naomi Remen, M.D.,
KITCHEN TABLE WISDOM

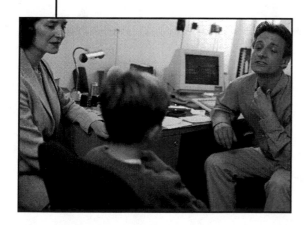

Imagine this from the patient's perspective: a female patient has been waiting for her male physician for 20 minutes. She is angry at his tardiness, in addition to being in pain and worried about her symptoms. The physician walks into the room, looks at his watch, and looks down his nose over his reading glasses as the patient describes her symptoms. He then crosses his arms and interrupts the patient 20 seconds into her discussion about the nature of her pain.

On a scale of 1–10, how comfortable would this patient be talking to her physician? How much confidence would this patient have that the physician is really listening and paying attention to what she is saying? How much like an equal partner would this patient feel in her health care? And what, if anything, should the physician have done differently?

According to Geri Amori, Ph.D., CPHRM, ARM, director of the Professional Development and Education Center at the Risk Management and Patient Safety Institute, the physician in this scenario should have done the following:

- Apologized for being late (as a sign of respect for the patient's time)
- Not looked at his watch (so as not to seem in a hurry)
- Taken off his reading glasses (so as not to look down his nose at the patient)
- Sat down to meet the patient at eye level (to convey both interest and equality)
- Uncrossed his arms (which would have conveyed openness to what the patient had to say)

Each clinician-patient encounter is an opportunity for both parties to communicate, that is, to speak, to listen, to understand, and to respond appropriately to what the other has just said. Communication is the foundation for developing rapport and partnership.[1] It is essential for patient satisfaction and patient safety. Yet, on average, clinicians listen to their patients for 18 to 23 seconds before interrupting.[2] The act of interrupting accomplishes at

On average, clinicians listen to their patients for 18 to 23 seconds before interrupting.

least three things: (1) it stops the flow of information, increasing the chances the clinician will miss something important that the patient would have revealed if allowed a little more time to speak; (2) it increases the likelihood of the patient ending the clinical interview with the phrase, "Oh, by the way doctor," also known as the "doorknob question"[3]; and (3) interrupting the patient stops the two-way communication that a relationship needs to develop.[2] This chapter focuses on achieving effective, complete, and purposeful two-way communication between clinicians and patients in every encounter.

Helping Patients Speak Up

The strategies clinicians should use to communicate effectively with their patients will differ from one patient to another, according to Amori, because "One size does not fit all." Clinicians may need to let some patients speak until they're finished; gently guide others who tend to ramble to focus on their main problem; or question and read the patient's body language to elicit information when none is forthcoming.

Putting Patients at Ease

Patients will be comfortable sharing their personal and medical histories and other potentially important information most readily if they feel at ease with their clinicians.[2,4,5] Patients are put at ease when clinicians convey warmth, understanding, and confidence in their patients and when clinicians let patients know that their participation in their care is both welcome and invited.[4,6] All the information that the patient discusses—whether related to symptoms, medical history, potential adverse reactions to medication, or concerns about the potential for medical errors—is potentially important. Clinicians can put patients at ease by letting them know that no question is too trivial and no piece of information is too minor to share.[5]

> **Tip**
>
> Patients will have different abilities and desires to partner in their care. Clinicians should, therefore, begin by asking patients questions such as the following:
>
> - How would you like to participate in your care?
>
> - It's your body and your health. My job is to help you achieve the best health for you. How are we going to partner, how are we going to do this together?
>
> —Geri Amori, Ph.D., CPHRM, ARM, director of the Professional Development and Education Center at the Risk Management and Patient Safety Institute

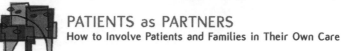
Clinicians often believe that doing what is required to put patients at ease will take time they cannot afford; but an investment of several minutes initially will yield dividends later, leading to clinicians' thorough understanding of the patient's problems,[3] patients' greater cooperation with treatment, fewer follow-up visits and telephone calls, and reduced potential for errors.

Consider this: "If the doctor lets the patient go on for three to four minutes, they tell you 90% of what's wrong with them."[2] Still, letting patients go on is no guarantee that they will reveal their most worrisome problems either first or even after three or four minutes. "If the most bothersome symptom is biomedical, it will probably not be voiced first about 50% of the time. If the chief symptom is psychosocial, it is even less likely to come up first."[3] It isn't enough for clinicians to listen without interruption; they also need to set the agenda for the interview by asking patients questions meant to elicit all of the patient's concerns...before the caregiver puts his or her hand on the doorknob.[3]

Strategies for Initiating Conversations with Patients

Clinicians should ask themselves five questions to help them set the agenda for each visit[3]:

1. What are the patient's primary concerns for this visit?
2. What are the clinician's concerns about the patient?
3. What are the patient's specific requests?
4. Which of the patient's requests or clinician's concerns should be addressed today, and which can be addressed in subsequent visits?
5. What disagreements about priorities exist between patient and clinician, and how can these be negotiated?

Clinicians could ask patients the following questions at the beginning of each visit[3]:

- What brings you in today?
- What kinds of problems are concerning you today?

- What else did you want to discuss today?
- Other than these problems, what else did you want to be sure we begin to discuss today?
- What else do you need to have taken care of today?

The strategies clinicians should use to initiate conversations with patients will depend on the patient, according to Amori. To draw patients out, Amori encourages clinicians to make statements or ask questions such as the following:

- "I know you have a lot of thoughts about this."
- "How will this treatment affect your life?"
- "I know you must have questions."
- "What are you unsure about?"
- "What can I make clearer?"
- "How might this be a problem for you?"

"If a patient is rambling," Amori says, "the clinician can gently ask, 'If you had only one sentence to explain your concerns, what would that be?'"

Patients who accept what the clinician says too readily, who ask no questions, or who look as if they are not paying attention show signs that they don't really understand what the clinician has said, Amori says. It is important for clinicians to ask questions that will help them determine whether patients have heard, understood, and agreed with what they have just said. Asking questions that require patients to repeat back what the clinician has just said in their own words—that is, using the "teach-back" method—is more effective than asking questions to which the answer is a simple "yes" or "no." Instead of asking patients if they understand how to take their medications, physicians should ask how they *plan* to take their medication in the course of their day. Clinicians should explain why a medication is important, mention any adverse reactions to watch out for, and tell patients how and when they should take their medication. Patients will not necessarily take their medication just because their physician tells them to, Amori cautions, which is why discussions need to be as interactive as possible.

"If the doctor lets the patient go on for three to four minutes, they tell you 90% of what's wrong with them."

Strategies for Continuing Conversations

Before focusing on the first problem the patient mentions, it is important to know all the patient's concerns.[3] A complete understanding will allow the clinician to set priorities for each visit, negotiate with the patient what will be attended to first, and set the agenda for subsequent visits.[3] Gathering as much information from the patient as possible will reduce the likelihood of the patient's leaving potentially important concerns unexpressed and unresolved.[3] To elicit more information from a patient or to clarify answers that are unclear or incomplete, clinicians should ask questions such the following[3,8]:

Probing Questions

- What else would you like to talk about today?
- Is there anything more you'd like to talk about?
- What specific requests do you have today, such as . . . ?
- Is there a specific question I might be able to answer for you right now, or should we set aside more time to discuss that at another visit?

Communicating over the Telephone

Communicating with patients by telephone presents its own set of challenges. Unlike the situation in a face-to-face visit, clinicians may not be aware that, when they call, their patients are not alone—and in that case may be less than forthcoming about their symptoms or concerns. When patients call during the night requesting a prescription for narcotics, physicians have no access to medical records that would help them determine the legitimacy of such requests. Patients may be reluctant to state the real reason for their late-night phone calls because they fear "disturbing" the physician. Patients who call may be hearing impaired, not speak English well, have noise in the background, have a bad connection, or all of the above.[7]

To overcome these challenges, Anna B. Reisman and colleagues recommend using approaches including, but not limited to, the following[7]:

- Let patients know during their office visit how test results will be communicated.

- When calling with a test result, ask if the patient can speak freely.

- Do not leave test results with family members without specific permission from the patient to do so, and do not leave results on answering machines.

- Be cautious about interpreting information provided by others.

SIDEBAR 2.1

- Always speak with the patient directly.

- Establish policies about prescribing narcotics or other medication over the phone and make patients aware of these policies through "controlled substance contracts."

- When it is difficult to deny a patient's telephone request, use phrases that convey empathy and warmth, such as, "I wish I could, but. . . ."

- Ask patients to repeat back instructions to ensure their understanding.

- Notice the patient's tone of voice, pitch, pauses, and any other clues as to whether the patient might need emergency care.

- Allow patients time to describe their primary complaint before interrupting.

- After patients have described their primary complaint, ask, "Is there anything else you want me to know about?"

- Be honest about difficulties understanding the patient.

- Use simple statements and direct questions, summarize often, and check with the patient to confirm understanding.

- Ask whether a family member can translate. ∎

- What else can you tell me about that?
- What has this been like for you?
- Is this all right with you?

Seeking Clarification
- Let me see if I understand. . . .
- What I'm hearing you say is . . .
- Will you correct me if I haven't gotten this right?

Responding to Patient Concerns
- That sounds very difficult.
- I can imagine that this might feel . . .
- I can see that you are . . .
- You must feel good about that.

At the very least, clinicians should encourage patients to understand the answers to three questions[9]:

1. What is your main problem?
2. What do you need to do? and
3. Why is it important for you to do this?

Just as clinicians can observe, according to Amori, that patients do not always understand or listen, patients believe that clinicians neither listen to nor understand their problems.[3] Clinicians, therefore, must not only ensure that patients are listening and understanding, but demonstrate to patients that they have both listened and understood.[3]

Pausing several seconds after patients have answered each of the clinician's questions can help patients feel understood, respected, and taken seriously.[8]

"It may be helpful to remember," Amori suggests, "that even adult patients who under ordinary circumstances are forthcoming, generally well informed, and want to participate actively in their health care can find communication difficult when they are afraid, vulnerable, in unfamiliar surroundings, and trying to understand terms they have never heard before." All patients, therefore, can benefit from clinicians' help to communicate effectively.

Strategies for Asking About Pain

Asking patients questions about their pain and how they would describe it can yield important information when patients aren't sure how to communicate their pain clearly. Because pain can't be measured objectively, clinicians must rely on the patient's descriptions to treat it effectively. If patients are unable to describe their pain precisely, clinicians should help them by asking questions such as the following:

- When did the pain start?
- Where is it located?
- What makes it feel better or worse?
- Does it spread to another area?
- How does it feel now?
- How does it feel at its worst?
- How does it feel at its best?
- How would you rate the pain on a scale of 1 to 10?
- What do you think caused your pain?
- What methods of relief have you tried, with what results?
- How is the pain affecting your life?

Asking patients to describe their pain by using adjectives such as stabbing, aching, dull, tingling, or throbbing will also aid the clinician's understanding.[10]

"When the family is there, address the family—say something like, 'When your loved one is ill, we'll try to make you aware of what's going on, what medications are being given, and so on.'"

Strategies for Communicating with Adolescents

Communicating with adolescents poses special challenges. Because adolescents do not disclose information readily, are afraid of being judged, want to be spoken to directly, and are concerned about confidentiality, it is especially important for clinicians to reassure them that everything they discuss is confidential.[4] Of all age groups, adolescents are the least likely to receive medical care—including prenatal care—and typically engage in high-risk behaviors.[4] It is important when treating adolescents, particularly females, to be comforting and understanding of the patient's needs and to explain medical procedures fully.[4] (For more information about involving adolescents in their care, *see* Chapter 5, "Addressing the Education and Involvement Needs of Special Populations.")

 Use the "teach-back" method to assess patients' understanding of their conditions, prescribed medications, upcoming procedures, and so on. Carefully word your question so that it requires the patient to explain his or her understanding rather than simply answer "yes" or "no."

Communicating with Patient Representatives

Just as clinicians should respect and put patients at ease, they should respect and put family members at ease, thereby encouraging them to be part of the health care team. As Amori advises, "When the family is there, address the family—say something like, 'When your loved one is ill, we'll try to make you aware of what's going on, what medications are being given, and so on. Please call our attention to anything that looks wrong to you, such as a bag hanging crookedly or anything at all.'"

If a family member or other patient representative tries to speak for the patient—unless the patient is too groggy to speak—Amori advises the clinician to gently say something like, "First let me talk with Mom—then we can talk, too." If the patient is too groggy to speak, the clinician can then talk with the patient's representative.

If a family member or other patient representative would like to stay in the patient's room during an examination to take notes, the clinician should first ask whether this is all right with the patient.[11]

"Clinicians need to remember," says Amori, "patients are scared, mistrustful of doctors and hospitals, and they feel helpless. They are in foreign environments. Under these circumstances people are not usually at their best. It's important to be understanding."

Effectively Communicating About Medical Errors

The most difficult conversation for clinicians to have with patients and their families may be the one they must have after an unintended adverse outcome has occurred. According to the Risk Management Foundation, "Caregivers have historically held back from talking openly with patients about medical mistakes because they are concerned about the legal implications. However, recent research and growing interest from organized medicine and patient advocacy groups is beginning to change that position."[13] In fact, one of the reasons many patients and their families sue for malpractice is that they are angry that medical organizations and physicians did not talk with them about what happened in a clear, straightforward way.[13]

"Many people harmed by their treatment suffer further trauma through the incident being insensitively and inadequately handled.

"Patients and families don't want to hear how errors happen in general— they want to hear how this particular error happened."

SIDEBAR 2.2

Humor Dispensed with Caution

Humor can play a role throughout patient–provider communication, but it must be used with extreme caution and sensitivity because it can easily cause offense. Before attempting to use humor, Amori advises, clinicians and patients first must establish a relationship of mutual trust, understanding, and friendship. Clinicians need to learn whether a patient appreciates humor and gauge the mood of the patient at each visit. If a child is ill or the parent is distressed or angry, for example, clinicians should not use humor.[12] Under the right circumstances, laughter can be therapeutic, especially with children—laughter can relieve tension and can help children overcome their fear of seeing the doctor.[12]

When used in the right place, at the right time, and in the right way, humor can help clinicians open lines of communication, perhaps making it easier for patients to discuss difficult issues. But the potential for humor to have unintended negative consequences is great and therefore must be attempted only with the utmost care, sensitivity, and skill.[12] ■

Conversely, when the staff comes forward, acknowledges the damage, and takes the necessary action, the overall impact can be greatly reduced. Injured patients need an explanation and an apology to know that changes have been made to prevent future incidents, and these patients often also need practical and financial help. The absence of any of these factors can be a powerful stimulus to a complaint or litigation."[6]

Ilene Corina, copresident of Persons United Limiting Substandards and Errors (PULSE), agrees. If an error occurs, Corina advises the attending physician "to have an honest, open, compassionate conversation with the patient, family, or both as soon as possible. Patients and their families want and deserve to know what happened." In many cases, disclosing the causes of an unanticipated adverse outcome will take place during more than one conversation, as the reasons for such an outcome become clear. Corina advises physicians to talk to patients and their families as if they're talking to their own mother, other family members, or friends. She also recommends that a trained layperson, such as a social worker or a chaplain, be present when the physician explains a medical error to be sure the explanation is clear and understandable. "Patients and families," she says, "don't want to hear how errors happen in general—they want to hear how this particular error happened."

> ## JOINT COMMISSION STANDARD
>
> **RI.2.90** Patients and, when appropriate, their families are informed about the outcomes of care, treatment, and services that have been provided, including unanticipated outcomes.

"Real explanations diffuse anger in families," Corina says. "Patients and families are angry when physicians do not talk to them, or when physicians talk to them in ways that are not real, genuine, or honest. Patients and their families know when they're being told the truth and when they're being lied to," she says, "and they want the physician and the organization to take responsibility for an error and apologize for it."

Lucian Leape, M.D., coauthor of the 1999 Institute of Medicine report *To Err Is Human,* said at a 2005 conference in sessions focusing on "The Power of Apology," "Legal concerns aren't the only barrier to apology. Obstacles include the emotional challenge of apologizing, a lack of awareness of how silence impacts patients, and a lack of communication skills."[13]

A proper apology is an essential part of good care after a patient is harmed, according to Leape, and must include the following four essential elements[13]:

1. Acknowledge the event.
2. Explain what caused the error.
3. Show remorse.
4. Make amends.

Perhaps at no time is having established a good relationship with a patient more important for the clinician than when an error must be disclosed, Corina notes. "A relationship between a physician and a patient should be established long before disclosure. But if someone with whom the patient and family have no relationship, such as an anesthesiologist, must disclose an error, disclosure should be handled with the utmost honesty and compassion," she says.

Tip Have a social worker or chaplain present with the physician when explaining the medical error to a patient and his or her family.

There is no standard or ideal way to disclose medical errors and no guarantee of the legal outcome after disclosure. According to Corina, the purpose of disclosure is not to protect the physician or the organization; rather, disclosure helps patients and their families begin the long and difficult process of grieving; it helps them decide what they will do next; and, as in the case of the Dana-Farber Cancer Institute described in Chapter 1, full disclosure helps medical organizations understand what went wrong and what needs to be done to prevent such errors from recurring in their institutions.

Unlike patients who have experienced medical errors firsthand, many people may feel medical errors won't happen to them or to their family members. And even if they are concerned, patients and their families may not know they can play a vital role in medical error prevention. Chapter 3 highlights the pivotal role of medical organizations, clinicians, and the media in raising public awareness of medical error prevention and in empowering everyone to become attentive and assertive partners in their health care.

References

1. Cleaveland C.: *Sacred Space: Stories from a Life in Medicine.* Philadelphia: American College of Physicians, 1998.

2. Belzer E.J.: Improving patient communication in no time. *Family Practice Management* May 1999. http://www.aafp.org/fmp/990500fm/23.html (accessed Sep. 21, 2005).

3. Baker L.H., O'Connell D., Platt F.W.: "What else?" Setting the agenda for the clinical interview. *Ann Intern Med* 143:766–770, Nov. 15, 2005.

4. Clowers M.: Young women describe the ideal physician. *Adolescence* 37:695–704, Winter 1992.

5. Meyer G.S., Arnheim L.: The power of two: Improving patient safety through better physician-patient communication. *Fam Pract Manag* 9:47–48, Jul.–Aug. 2002.

6. Vincent C.A., et al.: Patient safety: What about the patient? http://www.qualityhealthcare.com, downloaded from http://qhc.bmjjournals.com (accessed Aug. 29, 2005).

7. Reisman A.B., Brown K.E.: Preventing communication errors in telephone medicine: A case-based approach. *J Gen Intern Med* 20:959–963, Oct. 2005.

8. Coulehan J.L., et al.: "Let me see if I have this right...": Words that help build empathy. *Ann Intern Med* 135:221–227, Aug. 7, 2001.

9. Partnership for Clear Health Communication: *What Is Ask Me Three?* http://www.askme3.org (accessed Dec. 9, 2005).

10. Singer B.W.: I feel your pain: Patient-physician communication and drug use in treatment of pain. *Better Homes & Gardens.* http://www.findarticles.com (accessed Aug. 26, 2005).

11. Chronic Conditions Information Network (CCIN): *Be a Friend with a Pen.* Cavendish, VT: CCIN, 2005. http://www.cc-info.net (accessed Oct. 21, 2005).

12. Bennett H.J.: Humor in Medicine. *South Med J* 96:1257–1261, Dec. 2003.

13. Risk Management Foundation: *Time Has Come to Apologize.* http://www.rmf.harvard.edu/patientsafety/apology_lecture_post.asp (accessed Dec. 9, 2005)

"A relationship between a physician and a patient should be established long before disclosure."

PATIENT PERSPECTIVE 2.1
ROXANNE GOELTZ'S STRUGGLE TO BE A PARTNER IN HER CARE

When a patient feels mistrustful and afraid of medical institutions and physicians yet wants to participate fully in his or her health care, not being able to do so may be frustrating, demoralizing, and anxiety provoking. This is Roxanne Goeltz's story.

Roxanne Goeltz's brother, Mike, died in September 1999 from what the family believed was a medical error but for which they did not sue. In February 2000 she and her son experienced stuffiness and earaches, and they reluctantly sought medical attention. "That visit did nothing to reassure me," Goeltz says. "There was no real interaction with the doctor. We sat; he listened to our symptoms, prescribed some pills to dry up our congestion, and then sent us on our way. Nothing made me feel like a partner. I took the prescriptions, had them filled, and started taking them without really paying attention to what we were taking or why."

"There was no real interaction with the doctor. . . . Nothing made me feel like a partner."

She returned to the clinic in May 2000 when she experienced dizziness and a variety of other symptoms. She thought she might be suffering from depression, so she made up her mind to talk to whomever she saw at the clinic first. Although the health care worker was responsive and seemed interested, her body language and manner conveyed that she did not have much time to listen. Goeltz did not want to impose, so gave her a hurried explanation of her symptoms. She was told to "give it three more weeks."

"I couldn't wait," Goeltz says. "Internally, I was in sheer panic that there was something horribly wrong with me. I'd done some research on the Internet and came up with several possibilities. I had to find someone who would listen, so I called the nurse line that is available through my insurance. She was patient, listened to my symptoms, and suggested that I make an appointment with

PATIENT PERSPECTIVE 2.1

my doctor to be examined. When I told her my only doctor was a gynecologist, she recommended that I give that office a call. When I did so, the person who answered the telephone chastised me. To quote: 'Doctor does not see patients. Call another department.' She then ended the call, without any referrals or suggestions about where to find a different doctor. . . . I realized that I had to take the initiative. It was my health and well-being at stake and I had a responsibility to take care of myself."

Goeltz called the clinic again and made an appointment with the first internal medicine specialist who had an opening. "I will never forget this doctor for as long as I live," she said. "When I talked to him, I felt like I was stepping off a steep cliff. He not only caught me, but also in his words and manner encouraged me to keep jumping off each cliff I came to: I believed he would be there to support me. I shared all my symptoms, Mike's story, my fear of being written off as depressed, and my worry that depression was masking real physical problems. He listened without rushing me, calmly writing notes. He thought about what I had to say, and encouraged me to say more. I felt like he was pulling out of me the information I so wanted to discuss with someone who had expertise to help me decipher what was going on. We parted that day with a series of tests set up and a plan to look at the possibility of depression if the tests indicated I was sound physically. He asked me if I was in agreement with the route he had mapped out. I left there feeling much better about the health care system in general and remember thinking that maybe some of them did care and could be trusted. Although I didn't put it together at that moment, it was the beginning of partnering with my doctor!"

In Goeltz's words, "One of the tests—a chest x-ray—identified a problem. The doctor had ordered it because I reported being short of breath, a symptom I was initially hesitant to reveal because I thought it was related to the weight I'd gained and I was embarrassed! It was the doctor's respect for me and my resulting trust in him that encouraged me to share this vital

"He listened without rushing me, calmly writing notes. . . . I felt like he was pulling out of me the information I so wanted to discuss with someone who had expertise to help me decipher what was going on."

PATIENT PERSPECTIVE 2.1

piece of information. The x-ray came back showing a small shadow by my lungs, which prompted a CT scan identifying a mass in my chest.

"My next appointment was with the cardiothoracic surgeon, during which I thought he was to do a biopsy of the mass to determine if it was cancer. . . . The first impression made by the surgeon was one of a gentle confidence, and our communication was an extraordinary example of what it means to be partners.

"I was anxious to know whether the mass was cancer, and really wanted the biopsy that I was expecting done. He disagreed. But, rather than discounting my wishes or telling me what to do, he fully explained his rationale. The location and size of the mass next to my vital organs required it to be removed, in his opinion, whether or not it was cancer. He advised that doing a biopsy and a subsequent surgery would put me through an unnecessary procedure, but he left it up to me to decide what I wanted to do. In that one episode of communication, I knew he was a person who respected and was listening to me. I felt I could share all my feelings and concerns with him, and I did. I made the decision to follow his advice before our appointment was over, and said, 'Let's take it out. I am ready. I have not eaten since before midnight, so let's do it now!'

"He laughed and told me that things do not happen that quickly. He was going on vacation for two weeks and we could schedule it after that, but I said, 'No, I have just shared my most personal feelings and fears with you. I trust and want you to do the surgery.' He looked at me for a few seconds. I felt just as confident as he seemed to be. Then he smiled and invited me to go with him to see his scheduler. I had surgery two days later, before he went on vacation!

"While I was satisfied with myself for how I dealt with this surgeon, I must say that it only happened because he allowed it to happen. He partnered with me at the level I wanted and was

PATIENT PERSPECTIVE 2.1

capable of handling. He also invited me to call him if I had further concerns. I did so, the night before surgery, as I was experiencing very cold feet. He responded to my page quickly, listened to my being nervous, and was very reassuring. I relaxed and thanked him, confident that the decision he helped me reach was the right one for me."

But Goeltz's positive experience with her surgeon was far different from her experience with her new oncologist. In her words, "In the hospital, now recovering from both chest surgery and an embolism, the oncologist who was assigned to me greeted me for the first time by saying, 'I was elected to come talk to you.' He then told me I had a malignant thymoma. I was alone. When I heard the word *malignant,* I shut out everything that came after it and began crying. The oncologist was impatient and asked what I was crying about. I told him I was upset because he had just told me I had cancer. He said he had not. What ensued could only be described as an argument. Shortly into it, the oncologist threw up his hands, said he would have someone else talk to me in the morning, and walked out.

"After my surgeries and radiation treatments, I had two follow-up appointments with the oncologist. I wanted to work with him and hoped that if we met under less stressful circumstances we could communicate. I brought information to our appointments I'd gathered through my own research to help establish my follow-up care plan. I truly believe I gave him the chance to work with me, but after two appointments I knew I had to trade him in. He would not discuss the studies I brought with me or address any of my concerns, saying they were unimportant. His treatment plan was vague and he relayed it to me in a condescending manner. I had no say in what kind of protocol would be used for follow-up monitoring and care." Goeltz found another oncologist with whom she could work in true partnership.

Source: Goeltz R., et al.: Trial and error in my quest to be a partner in my health care: A patient's story. In Youngberg B.J., Hatlie M.J. (eds.): *The Patient Safety Handbook.* Sudbury, MA: Jones and Bartlett, 2004.

CHAPTER THREE
Persuading and Teaching Patients to Get Involved

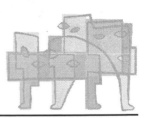

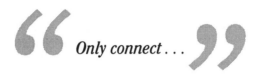

Only connect . . .

E.M. Forster,
HOWARD'S END

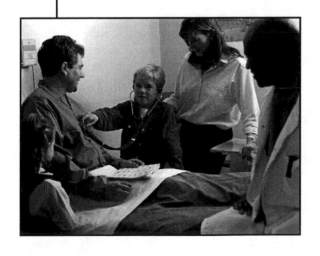

When reports of medical errors make the news, the stories can be as shocking and unforgettable as reports of airplane crashes. The 1994 medical error at the Dana-Farber Cancer Institute that resulted in the death of *Boston Globe* reporter Betsy Lehman and the permanent injury of Maureen Bateman became the focus of intense and ongoing media scrutiny (*see* Chapter 1 for more information about this case). The media shine their spotlight on wrong-site surgery, anesthesia accidents, medication errors, and more. Layered on top of such stories is the statistic that more than two in five, or 42%, of adults' lives have been touched by a medical error in some way.[1]

More than two in five, or 42%, of adults' lives have been touched by a medical error in some way.

The many causes of medical errors and the means to prevent them, including the role that patients and their families can play, may not be the primary message in media accounts. To create public awareness about *patient safety* as opposed to medical errors, and the role that each person can play in maintaining it, some medical institutions, such as Gettysburg Hospital, in Gettysburg, Pennsylvania, contribute columns to their local newspapers. But despite such efforts, are members of the general public aware that up to 70% of medical errors are preventable, and that they themselves can play a crucial role in their prevention?[1] The answer, apparently, is "no": Despite media coverage not only of medical errors but of changes that health care organizations have made as a result, and despite the efforts of many organizations to disseminate information about the essential role every individual can play in preventing errors, not everyone seems to be aware that they themselves can make health care safer.[1] And many of those who are aware apparently still feel uncomfortable asking their clinicians questions they perceive to be challenging, such as "Have you washed your hands?"[1]

To complicate matters, it is unclear whether, despite ongoing public education efforts, the general public really understands what the term *patient safety* means.[1] Against this backdrop of attempts to educate the public with less than optimal results, how can institutions, organizations, and clinicians increase patients' and others' awareness of medical errors and encourage their active participation to make health care safer? And how can they use the media to do so? This chapter explains how some organizations have gone about it.

Campaigns to Help Prevent Medical Errors

If organizations and clinicians can persuade people that they actual-ly *can* prevent medical errors while being given simple, clear instructions about how to do so, patients and their families are like-ly to believe they can make a difference and to act on that belief.[1] Several public education campaigns are taking this approach.

Since March 2002, the Joint Commission and the Centers for Medicare & Medicaid Services have sponsored the "Speak Up" cam-paign to forge partnerships among medical organizations, health care professionals, and health care consumers in an effort to reduce medical errors. The Speak Up campaign encourages health care consumers to actively participate in their care and empowers them with the tools to do so. The information is written in English and Spanish and explains how to help ensure the patient's safety throughout medications, diagnosis, testing, surgery, and other top-ics. The Speak Up campaign encourages all health care consumers to take the following actions[2]:

- **S**peak up if you have questions or concerns, and if you don't understand, ask again. It's your body and you have a right to know.
- **P**ay attention to the care you are receiving. Make sure you're get-ting the right treatments and medications by the right health care professionals. Don't assume anything.
- **E**ducate yourself about your diagnosis, the medical tests you are undergoing, and your treatment plan.
- **A**sk a trusted family member or friend to be your advocate.
- **K**now what medications you take and why you take them. Medication errors are the most common health care errors.
- **U**se a hospital, clinic, surgery center, or other type of health care organization that has undergone a rigorous on-site evaluation against established state-of-the-art quality and safety standards, such as that provided by the Joint Commission.
- **P**articipate in all decisions about your treatment. You are the center of the health care team.

The "Speak Up" campaign encourages health care consumers to actively participate in their care and empowers them with the tools to do so.

Another well-established public education campaign is "Talk About Prescriptions Month," an annual campaign sponsored by the National Council on Patient Information and Education. The goal of this campaign is to increase consumer awareness of the importance of being actively involved to prevent medication errors. The council's latest effort, "The 3 Rs for Safe Medicine Use," focuses on consumer awareness of Risk, Respect, and Responsibility[3]:

Risk—Recognize that all medicines (prescription and nonprescription) have risks as well as benefits, and you need to weigh these risks and benefits carefully for every medicine you take.

Respect—Respect the power of your medicine and the value of medicines properly used.

Responsibility—Take responsibility for learning about how to take each medication safely. Being responsible also means following this important rule: When in doubt, ask first. Your health care professional can help you get the facts you need to use medicines correctly.

> *Tip* To disseminate these empowering messages, heath care organizations can print "Speak Up" materials for patient rooms; sponsor local public service announcements using their own physicians and nurses; include the brochure content in patient information materials, Web sites, and community newsletters; distribute material at health fairs; share it on closed-circuit patient education television; use it for staff education and orientation; and distribute it through bedside tent cards.[2]

To reduce wrong-site surgery by educating patients and encouraging them to take an active role in its prevention, the American Academy of Orthopaedic Surgeons launched the "Sign Your Site" campaign in 1997.* As part of this effort, the patient's surgical and health care teams gave patients information and explicit instructions on how they could help to prevent wrong-site surgery. (The Joint Commission had identified one of the underlying causes of wrong-site surgery as the breakdown in communication between members of the surgical team and patients and their families.) Despite this campaign and the Joint Commission's efforts in working with health care organizations to help prevent wrong-site surgery,[4] many patients still believe that wrong-site

---

* The Joint Commission does not encourage having the patient mark the site; instead, it prefers that the person conducting the procedure mark the site with the active involvement of the patient.

surgery is so rare that it is unlikely ever to happen to them. The result of this attitude may be passivity on the part of patients and their families. The best way to counter these attitudes and change patient behavior is for surgeons and other members of the health care team to continue to strongly encourage patients and their families to take an active role in preparing for surgery.[5]

What happens as a result of these organization's campaigns depends on institutions and individual clinicians championing their causes. When patients and their families are educated and understand why and how they need to actively participate in their care, and when they feel empowered to do so, their involvement can help to prevent medical errors and enhance patient safety.

Educating and Empowering Patients

Preventing Medication Errors

Patients play an important role in the area of medication safety. Because drug-related mistakes are the most common kind of medical error, the health care industry needs patients to take an active role in managing their medications. Caregivers can encourage active participation at several steps in the process.

> **Tip** The National Council on Patient Information and Education supplies an array of materials to help organizations work with the media in educating the public about their role in preventing medication errors, including the following[3]:
>
> • Campaign background information
>
> • A planning kit
>
> • Tips for a successful campaign
>
> • Lists of questions health care consumers can ask when they get a new prescription medication and when the medication they are taking is in the news
>
> • Scripts for print and radio public service announcements, press releases, and posters advertising the campaign

When prescribing a new medication, physicians should always educate the patient about the drug's purpose and intended benefits. This practice, which is part of the informed consent and medication adherence process, can empower the patient to be a more effective participant in drug safety. In addition, physicians should do the following[6, 7]:

• Describe (and provide written information on) possible side effects. Patients and family members are the "first line of defense" in monitoring for adverse reactions.

- Explain what other medications, dietary supplements, food, drinks, or activities the patient should avoid while taking the medication.
- Make sure the patient can read the handwriting on the prescription.
- Write the reason for the medication on the prescription.
- Tell the patient when and for how long to take the medication.
- Ask patients how they plan to fit taking the prescribed medication into their daily life.
- Describe how the patient should take the medication (for example, should the patient chew or swallow the medicine).
- Give patients and family members clear, easy-to-understand, scientifically accurate, and nonpromotional written information about the medication to take home. This information should only reiterate what was said during the office visit; it should not contain new information.

See *Case Study 3.1 on page 62 for more information about medication adherence and medication reconciliation.*

See *Case Study 3.1 on page 62 for more information about medication adherence and medication reconciliation.*

SIDEBAR 3.1

The Role of the Patient Advocate

According to Margo Caulfield, co-director of the Chronic Care Information Network of Vermont and New Hampshire (http://www.cc-info.net), a patient advocate is a critical member of the health care team, someone whom patients can count on to do the following:

- Accompany them to medical appointments, tests, treatments, and procedures.
- Ask specific questions.
- Take careful notes during each visit.
- Keep track of the medications the patient is taking.
- Go over their notes with the patient after the medical appointment to confirm or clarify information.
- Ensure that the patient's wishes are carried out when patients are unable to do so.
- Be a spokesperson for the entire family and a liaison with the health care team.

A patient advocate can be a responsible and trusted member of the patient's family or a friend; a professional, organization-affiliated Patient Advocate or Patient Representative; or a social worker, nurse, or chaplain.

If patients choose to involve a patient advocate in their care, members of the health care team should have the advocate's telephone number and should remind patients that their advocates should have the telephone numbers of the patient's health care providers, hospital, pharmacy, and people to contact in an emergency.[8]

"Advocacy training should be organized in all hospitals across the country," recommends Caulfield. The Chronic Care Information Network of Vermont and New Hampshire provides in-person training for using patient advocates through their "Train the Trainer" workshops, and provides materials for advocates, including "How to Be a Friend with a Pen." ■

When administering a medication, nurses and others can encourage patient involvement in several ways. These strategies enlist the patient in the team effort to guard against medication errors:

- Let the patient know what medication you are administering and how often he or she should receive it.
- Explain the medication's purpose and common side effects.
- When administering an IV, tell the patient how long the procedure should take.

- Explain patient-controlled analgesia devices to patients and family members and clarify who should and *who should not* push the button.
- When feasible, educate patients about the "five rights" of medication safety:
  1. Right patient
  2. Right medication
  3. Right time
  4. Right dose
  5. Right route

JOINT COMMISSION REQUIREMENT
Universal Protocol, Requirement 1B
Mark the operative site as described in the Universal Protocol (marking must take place with the patient involved, awake, and aware, if possible).

- Encourage patients to speak up if they think they are getting the wrong medications (or the wrong doses) or if they do not feel well after taking a medication.

Patient Identification
One of the key elements of medication safety is patient identification. Active patient involvement is essential to ensuring correct patient identity. To enhance this process, inform patients that caregivers should always check two forms of identification before administering a medication or blood product, taking blood samples, or providing any other treatment (National Patient Safety

Goal 1A). In addition, encourage patients to state their name and present their armband without being asked when they are approached with a medication.

Medication Reconciliation

In general, providers should encourage patients to maintain a list of their current medications (including prescriptions, over-the-counter drugs, supplements, and homeopathic remedies). Maintaining an up-to-date medication list is an effective way for patients to help physicians guard against adverse interactions and other potential problems. Organizations can support the process by reconciling a patient's medications upon entry (National Patient Safety Goal 8). Thereafter, the organization can provide patients with medication cards that include a list of all the medications they are taking and encourage them to continually update the card and carry it in their purses or wallets.

Organizations can find more information on medication reconciliation through the Massachusetts Coalition for the Prevention of Medical Errors (http://www.macoalition.org) and the Institute for Healthcare Improvement's "100,000 Lives Campaign," which includes medication reconciliation as one of its six initiatives for saving lives (http://www.ihi.org/IHI/Programs/Campaign).

Preventing Wrong-Site Surgery

Wrong-site surgery is an entirely preventable medical error; like preventing medication errors, preventing wrong-site surgery depends on the attentive, active participation of the patient, as well as the surgeon and other members of the health care team.[5] To empower patients to become involved, surgeons and other health professionals can encourage patients to take the following steps[4]:

- Discuss the surgery and make sure everyone involved agrees on exactly what will be done.
- Verify the information on identity bracelets and make sure any bracelets containing incorrect information are replaced immediately.
- Make sure the operative permit includes the correct information about the surgical site before signing.
- Read all medical forms thoroughly and really understand them before signing.
- Ask questions and keep asking until the answers are understood.
- Have a responsible family member or friend present at visits to the physician, surgeon, and hospital on the day of surgery.
- If possible, ask the patient or his or her family member to be involved in the process of marking the surgical site.

> **Tip** Think about the patient's perspective of patient identification. If the same nurse comes into the same patient's room three or four times a day to administer medications, and each time the nurse asks the patient's name and birth date, wouldn't the patient wonder why the nurse doesn't know the patient's name by now? It may give patients peace of mind to understand certain health care processes that may appear odd or confusing to them.

Other Methods of Teaching Patients to Get Involved

This chapter has focused on some of the ways in which public education campaigns can work through medical organizations to persuade clinicians and educate them to work in partnership with patients to reduce medical errors, specifically medication errors and wrong-site surgery. But there are many other areas in which clinicians should involve their patients as partners, including infection control and medical testing.

> **Tip** Improve the interviewing process with patients to find out what medications they are on. Prompt patients with open-ended, specific questions about their health as well as their medications. For example, go down the list of a patient's conditions, asking what medications he or she takes for each, or prompt the patient for medications prescribed by each of his or her physicians.

When it comes to infection control, the most important thing to do is to educate patients on the standards that should be followed in a health care setting:

- Inform patients that caregivers must always wash their hands (or use an alcohol-based hand rub) before providing care.

• Let patients know it is okay to ask caregivers whether they have washed their hands. (*See* Case Study 3.2 on page 67 for more information on involving patients in the hand hygiene process.)

As for medical testing, let patients know that they should never assume that "no news is good news" and that they should always check back on test results. Make sure the patient knows what phone number to call and when the results should be available. Clinicians should also encourage patients to ask if they don't understand why a test is being ordered and to keep asking until they understand and to ask questions about test results until they are clear.[7,8]

> **Tip** Take the time to explain any of your organization's safety procedures that might alarm the patient. For instance, if you ask an open-ended question such as "What are we operating on today?" the patient might think his or her caregivers don't know what is going on. Instead, explain that open-ended questions provide a safety mechanism for the health care team as it double-checks the patient's information with the organization's information. In addition, the surgeon or other members of the health care team could explain that they will be taking a time-out immediately before the procedure begins to verify they have the correct patient, correct site, and correct procedure and that this is a safety measure as well.

The more patients know about their illnesses or conditions, the better they will be able to take an active part in their care. By encouraging patients to educate themselves, health care organizations further strengthen the patient safety process. In addition to providing medical information directly to patients, consider compiling a list of Web sites that patients can visit for further background (*see* the Appendix for a list of resources to give to patients). Of course, individual caregivers cannot be expected to educate patients on the full spectrum of health and safety issues at every patient contact. Matthew Mireles, Ph.D., president and director of Research at the CRG Medical Foundation for Patient Safety, encourages health care organizations to develop safety checklists. Such checklists can include information points to communicate to patients at key moments in the care process.

But clinicians can't communicate with all patients by asking the same questions, using the same explanations, or using the same techniques. Ultimately, engaging patients as partners in their care will require multiple approaches and will happen in stages.[1] As helpful as the suggestions in this chapter may be, clinicians need to remember that all patients are different; have different language, literacy, and health literacy skills; and come from different cultures that can influence their ability to understand and participate actively in their care. Chapter 4 focuses on communicating with patients and families who need more help in understanding, agreeing to, and participating in their care.

References

1. Hibbard J.H., et al.: Can patients be part of the solution? Views on their role in preventing medical errors. *Med Care Res Rev* 62:601–616, Oct. 2005.

2. Joint Commission on Accreditation of Healthcare Organizations: *Speak Up: Help Prevent Errors in Your Care.* http://www.jcaho.org/accredited+organizations/speak+up/speak+up+index.htm (accessed Dec. 5, 2005).

3. National Council on Patient Information and Education: *Education Before You Medicate: "Talk About Prescriptions" Planning Kit for October 2005.* http://www.talkaboutrx.org/rxmonth2005_message.jsp (accessed Sep. 29, 2005).

4. Joint Commission on Accreditation of Healthcare Organizations: *Universal Protocol for Preventing Wrong Site, Wrong Procedure, Wrong Person Surgery.* http://www.jcaho.org/accredited+organizations/patient+safety/universal+protocol (accessed Dec. 5, 2005).

5. DiGiovanni C.W., Kang L., Manuel J.: Patient compliance in avoiding wrong-site surgery. *J Bone Joint Surg Am* 85:815–819, May 2003.

6. American Medical Association (AMA): *Guidelines for Physicians for Counseling Patients About Prescription Medications in the Ambulatory Setting.* Chicago: AMA, 2004.

7. Agency for Healthcare Research and Quality (AHRQ): *Your Medicine: Play It Safe.* Rockville, MD: AHRQ, 2003. http://www.ahrq.gov/consumer/safemeds/safemeds.htm (accessed Oct. 29, 2005).

8. National Patient Safety Foundation (NPSF): *The Role of the Patient Advocate.* McLean, VA: NPSF, 2003. http://www.npsf.org (accessed Oct. 13, 2005).

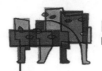
ARTICLE AT A GLANCE

Name of the organization:
Scripps Mercy Hospital is a private, not-for-profit hospital with two campuses located in San Diego, California. The 700-bed organization is part of a four-hospital system.

Purpose of the project:
Scripps Mercy Hospital wanted to improve patient education so patients would take their medication as recommended after hospital discharge.

Lessons learned:
Scripps Mercy learned that it is important to listen to patients because they provide a unique perspective on how to improve an organization's care, treatment, and services. Patients tended not to take their medications as prescribed before the project began, regardless of the patient's proficiency in English.

The Scripps Mercy Hospital staff also learned that changing human behavior can be challenging. By identifying people who could be champions for change, the organization was able to change the way the staff reconciled medications and educated patients.

Outcomes:
Scripps Mercy improved adherence to medication regimens among cardiac patients as a result of its new attempts to educate patients and reconcile medications. Following its success with cardiac patients, Scripps Mercy used these new methods elsewhere in the organization.

Staff involved:
Advanced practice nurse, nurse practitioner, cardiology director, medication reconciliation technician, director of pharmacy, chief of staff for the hospital, director of the cardiology catheterization lab, chief medical residents, internal medicine residents, nurse director of medicine and surgery, nurse educators, telemetry nurses, cardiology nurses, emergency department nurses, information systems staff, home health nursing staff.

CASE STUDY 3.1
IMPROVING MEDICATION ADHERENCE AT SCRIPPS MERCY HOSPITAL

Educating Patients About Their Medications

Patients who are involved in their own care are empowered to make educated health care decisions, understand and follow their treatment plan, discuss any concerns with their clinicians, and help to prevent medical errors.

As of January 2006, the Joint Commission will require disease-specific care, laboratories, and home care organizations to encourage the active involvement of patients and their families in the patient's own care, through National Patient Safety Goal 13. Although the Joint Commission made this goal applicable to a few select types of organizations, patient involvement is certainly relevant to all settings of care.*

Surveying Patients About Their Care

In 2002 Scripps Mercy Hospital embarked on a study to measure the postdischarge medication adherence of patients with cardiovascular disease. The organization wanted to determine whether the education provided to patients who were not proficient in English needed improvement. "Our hypothesis was

---

* The applicability of this goal is subject to change based on annual revisions to the National Patient Safety Goals. Please see *Joint Commission Perspectives* for the most up-to-date information on National Patient Safety Goals.

CASE STUDY 3.1

that patients who were proficient in English would have better adherence rates than patients who were not proficient in English," says David Shaw, M.D., director of medical education for Scripps Mercy.

The organization collected baseline data on 170 patients, equally split between English-proficient and non-English-proficient patients. "These people were taking an average of 10 medications that addressed a variety of comorbidities," says Shaw. Via a telephone survey, the organization asked each participant a series of questions about adherence to discharge medications. Patients were called 48 to 72 hours after discharge and again 30 days after discharge. The results of the baseline survey surprised the hospital. "What we discovered was that medication adherence in both groups was extremely poor, and, in fact, there was little difference between the adherence rates," says Shaw. "At 48 to 72 hours after discharge, both groups had about a 50% adherence rate. At 30 days, that rate dropped to 35%. The issue was not English proficiency, but medical literacy. We discovered that the way clinicians were giving information to patients was essentially like speaking to them in a foreign language."

As part of the baseline survey, Scripps Mercy queried patients on the problems with the education provided by the hospital. Patients identified the following three issues:

- In some cases, patients didn't understand what to do about their medications because verbal instructions were limited and there were no written instructions.
- In those cases where there were written instructions, they were either illegible or too complicated to understand. In many cases, medical terms were written in Latin.
- Clinicians failed to take into account patients' preadmission medications and how they would interact with postdischarge medications. "In some cases, because the patients had a longer relationship with the preadmission medications, they just went on taking those and skipped the new medications," says Shaw.

"The issue was not English proficiency, but medical literacy."

Implementing Initiatives to Improve Education

Based on these three issues, Scripps Mercy decided to improve their verbal education, written education, and medication reconciliation processes. An advanced practice nurse and a bilingual nurse practitioner implemented interventions on a test basis and monitored their success. In response to concerns about verbal education, the hospital designed and implemented a process in which the education was provided in the patient's preferred language, and medical terminology was avoided. Throughout the verbal education process, patients were asked if they understood the education provided, and caregivers were involved, when appropriate.

In response to patient feedback about written education, Scripps Mercy developed a computerized tool that provided clear, consistent, written education. This program included the following elements:

- Name of the medication
- Dosage
- Frequency
- When the medication should be taken
- Primary purpose of the medication
- Which preadmission medications to continue
- Which preadmission medications to modify in dose or frequency
- Which new medications to add
- Which preadmission medications to stop

All information printed from this computerized tool was in the patient's preferred language, and the information was written in a lower-grade reading level that was easy to understand.

Improving Medication Reconciliation

In addition to improving patient education, Scripps Mercy also worked with the staff to improve medication reconciliation.

CASE STUDY 3.1

The organization defined what to collect from patients and how to reconcile the patient's current medications with newly ordered medications. It emphasized the importance of reconciliation to the staff and monitored compliance.

Interventions Lead to Improvement

After Scripps Mercy revised its education and reconciliation processes, the hospital surveyed 85 cardiovascular patients. Again, the group was equally divided between English-proficient patients and those patients who were not proficient in English. "At 48 to 72 hours after discharge, patients receiving the education and reconciliation interventions had a 90% adherence to their medication regimen. At 30 days, there was 80% adherence," says Shaw. "As before, there was almost no difference between the English-proficient patients and those patients who were not proficient in English." The organization also monitored hospital readmissions and emergency department visits. Patients who received the education interventions did not have to visit the emergency department or be readmitted to the hospital because of noncompliance with medications, and overall hospitalizations were reduced by 40% within the six-month study period.

Applicable to More than Just Cardiac Patients

After Scripps Mercy determined that its new education initiatives were effective, it began rolling out the initiatives to the staff in different areas of internal medicine, such as diabetic care and renal care. To educate the staff about the new interventions, the organization provided in-services, created posters, and did demonstrations. "We did a marketing campaign of sorts, where we showed the staff how patient care could be improved, and we increased awareness about the importance of involving patients in their own care," says Shaw. The organization identified individuals who influenced other staff members and involved them in the training efforts.

"We did a marketing campaign of sorts, where we showed the staff how patient care could be improved, and we increased awareness about the importance of involving patients in their own care."

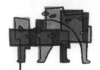

CASE STUDY 3.1

"We worked with champions of the process to help encourage the staff to move forward and change their behavior with regard to education and reconciliation," says Shaw.

The organization now uses the education and reconciliation interventions to help all internal medicine patients adhere to their medication regimens after discharge. "These processes could apply to any type of patients: pediatric patients, elderly patients, and anyone who takes multiple medications could benefit," says Shaw.

Continuing to Involve Patients

The hospital frequently updates the written education tool it created to make it more usable for the staff and patients. "We're currently pilot testing wallet cards created by the program that list all the patient's current prescriptions. We also are working to create a patient checklist that can be updated whenever patients visit a health care organization," says Shaw. Scripps Mercy continues to survey patients about their care to determine other ways the hospital could improve.

By educating patients about their medications and providing information that is clear and easy to understand, organizations of all types can involve patients in their own care and increase patient adherence to medication regimens.

Source: Joint Commission Resources: Case study: Improving medication adherence: Educating patients about their medications. *Patient Safety* 5:9–11, Nov. 2005.

CASE STUDY 3.2
HAVE YOU WASHED YOUR HANDS?

Implementing a Public Education Campaign to Empower Patients to Ask

Regular, frequent hand washing is the most effective strategy for preventing infection. But patients who may feel uncomfortable asking health care workers if they've washed their hands for fear of insulting them may be surprised to learn that health care workers wash their hands only 50% of the time. To empower patients to remind hospital staff to wash their hands routinely and to see what effect these reminders had on hand washing and infection rates, researcher and professor Maryanne McGuckin, Dr.Sc.Ed., developed the program *Partners in Your Care*.

Partners in Your Care consists of a brochure, video, and visual aids to encourage patients to remind hospital staff to wash their hands. Patients place a visual aid in their rooms in full view, which reminds staff to wash their hands even if patients are asleep or are otherwise unable to ask. Organizations that participate in the program receive a binder that includes a presentation agenda for the board of directors, brochures, measurement forms, and visual aids. Patients and their families are asked to read the brochure titled "Did You Wash Your Hands?" and to participate in the program. Any questions asked by patients or family members are answered by the hospital staff who provide direct patient care. If they can't answer patients' questions, then intensive care professionals are asked to help.

ARTICLE AT A GLANCE

Name of the organization:
Ingham Regional Medical Center, a subsidiary of McLaren Healthcare Corporation, is a community-based, university-affiliated teaching hospital in Lansing, Michigan, licensed for 400 patient beds.

Purpose of the project:
The *Partners in Your Care* program, developed by Maryanne McGuckin, Dr.Sc.Ed., at the University of Pennsylvania School of Medicine, produced a brochure, video, and visual aids to encourage patients and their families to ask health care workers if they have washed their hands, thereby helping to prevent infections.

Lessons learned:
Implementing a program such as this requires time to plan, to educate health care workers about its purpose, and to overcome any initial resistance.

Outcomes:
There are indications that asking health care workers whether they have washed their hands has played a role in increasing hand washing and decreasing infections.

Staff involved:
Infection control manager, finance department, environmental services department, nurses, physicians, patients, and families.

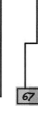

PATIENTS as PARTNERS
How to Involve Patients and Families in Their Own Care

CASE STUDY 3.2

The Ingham Regional Medical Center, in Lansing, Michigan, involved patients and their families in putting this program into practice in its cardiac intensive care unit and its surgical intensive care unit. In preparation, Ingham conducted extensive staff training to be sure staff wouldn't be insulted when patients asked whether they'd washed their hands. Not only did Ingham train its staff, but the organization also trained physicians who had privileges at the hospital but who were not employed there.

To evaluate this program's effectiveness, Ingham monitored the amount of hand soap and sanitizer used by the staff and tracked infection rates each month. Since this program began, there are indications that hand washing by staff has increased and infection rates have decreased.

Source: Joint Commission Resources: Case study: Ingham Regional Medical Center involves patients in the infection control process. *Patient Safety* 5:9–10, Apr. 2005.

Ingham

conducted

extensive

staff training

to be sure

staff wouldn't

be insulted

when patients

asked whether

they'd washed

their hands.

CHAPTER FOUR
Understanding Health Literacy
and Improving Informed Consent

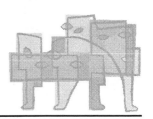

 Reading paperwork is like emotional

mountain-climbing for me. I would

rather walk 10 miles than to have to

read, understand, and sign 2 forms. At

least I know I can walk 10 miles.

Toni Cordell,
LITERACY ADVOCATE

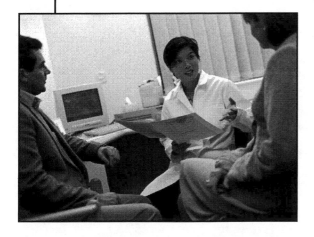

A Spanish-speaking woman walks out of the hospital just prior to surgery when it is finally communicated to her clearly that tubal ligation is a permanent sterilization technique, not a temporary method of birth control.[1]

A number of patients named a different side of the body or a different type of surgery than what was indicated on their charts when questioned just prior to surgery.[1]

Fortunately, these misunderstandings did not result in harm. But why did they occur? Presumably, the physicians explained these patients' conditions, discussed the risks and benefits of surgery and other options, agreed on a course of action with each patient, and signed forms documenting that the patients had understood and consented to the surgery. And, presumably, the patients understood what their physicians told them about their conditions, understood the risks and benefits of the surgery or procedure, knew the other options to the surgery or procedure, agreed with their physician on a course of action, and signed informed consent forms indicating that they understood and consented to the surgery or procedure. But, as the saying goes, "Never presume." This chapter examines why and how such misunderstandings take place and what can be done to prevent them in the future.

> ## JOINT COMMISSION STANDARD
>
> **RI.2.40** Informed consent is obtained.

Communication: It Takes Two

A common cause of patients' misunderstanding may be a failure to communicate on both sides: On the one hand, physicians often fail to realize that not all patients (1) understand medical jargon, (2) have reading skills that allow them to read or understand forms on their own, (3) understand the oral explanations their physicians provide, or (4) really understand what they have agreed to when they sign consent forms. On the other hand, patients may fail to tell physicians that they don't understand what they have read or heard, may not ask for help to interpret the required forms, and may not always ask questions that would

SIDEBAR 4.1

Who Understands and Who Doesn't?

It may be difficult to tell from outward appearances which patients have low literacy skills and which do not. Most of those with low literacy skills are white, native-born Americans; many are from ethnic and racial minorities. People with low literacy skills tend to be poor, less educated, and elderly, with physical and mental disabilities as well as multiple health problems.[23] But because demographic information doesn't necessarily tell the whole story, how can health care professionals tell whether patients have low literacy skills? There are certain common behaviors to look for[2]:

• Patients who tend to avoid situations that require them to read

• Patients who often "forget" reading glasses

• Patients who often have family or friends interpret information for them in the office or who bring written materials home to discuss with family members

• Patients who don't fill out forms completely, complete forms too quickly, agree with information too readily, appear easily distracted, or have a "glazed over" expression

• Patients who don't ask questions

• Patients who can't restate the information they've been given in their own words ∎

let physicians know that further explanation is needed. If the cause of patients' misunderstanding is the failure to communicate clearly and completely on both sides, then the solution must involve both sides. Because physicians have more authority to control the communication within the patient–provider relationship, it is up to physicians not only to communicate more clearly and simply with all patients, but to recognize that some patients need more, or different, types of communication to aid their understanding.

"You Just Don't Understand"

How can physicians tell who understands them and who doesn't, who has low literacy skills and who doesn't, and who would benefit if the physician used a different approach to communicating? This may not be so easy because many patients tend to be good at covering up their deficiencies, according to literacy advocate Toni Cordell. Consider these statistics:

• Almost half of all adult Americans have limited literacy skills or worse—they have trouble reading signs and using transportation schedules, let alone understanding clinicians' oral and written explanations of disease, treatment, procedures, or surgery.[3] "Understanding and filling out forms without help," Cordell says, "is an insurmountable task."

- The average patient on Medicaid reads at a 5th grade level. These patients may struggle to read appointment slips, prescriptions, medication labels, physicians' instructions, patient education materials, and forms.[2]
- The average American reads at an 8th or 9th grade level. Medical forms are written at even higher levels than this; therefore, the average American would have trouble reading and understanding forms documenting informed consent.[2]
- Even patients who have high literacy skills may have trouble reading and understanding complex, specialized medical terminology, especially when they are ill and grappling with unwelcome news and difficult choices.[2,3]

Even those who appear to understand the information

SIDEBAR 4.2

Avoiding Medical Jargon

The health of 90 million Americans, according to the National Quality Forum, is at risk because patients don't understand their physicians' orders. To help patients understand, the American Medical Association distributed 10,000 educational kits to physicians across the country in 2004, encouraging providers to use plain English instead of complex medical jargon. The kits also advised physicians to ask patients to repeat, in their own words, the information their physicians have conveyed (a process known as the "teach-back" method). In talking with their patients, physicians also are advised to look patients in the eye and to use visual aids when necessary.[1]

The following vignettes illustrate some of the reasons why it's important to use plain language instead of medical jargon:

- A contrast dye was ordered for a patient's CT scan when the patient was allergic to contrast. "No allergies" was noted on the admission orders. The allergy was noted on the medication administration record—but not on the Patient Care Kardex. The nurse asked the patient if he was allergic to "contrast," but the patient said "no." He did not realize that the term "contrast" referred to IV dye. The patient was started on the contrast infusion and only later reported the allergy.

SIDEBAR 4.2

- A physician called the spouse of an elderly patient to obtain consent for a percutaneous endoscopic gastrostomy tube insertion, and the spouse agreed. The next day, the daughter visited and complained that a PEG/feeding tube was against the family's wishes. Upon investigation, it became clear that the spouse did not understand what he agreed to was a feeding tube procedure.

These misunderstandings may have been avoided if lay terms had been used instead of medical terminology, or if the medical terminology had been defined for patients and their families. ■

being communicated may not truly understand: After agreeing to or receiving care, 18% to 45% of patients are unable to recall the major risks of surgery, many cannot answer basic questions about the services or procedures they agreed to receive, 44% do not know the exact nature of their operation, and at least 60% do not read or understand the information contained in informed consent forms, despite having signed them. Half of all patients don't understand what their physicians have told them.[2] Such patients are not truly informed about the choices they have made.[1]

Many patients tend to be good at covering up their deficiencies.

According to Candace Moore, "We have built an entire system based on the assumption that patients can read and understand complex materials."[3] Regardless of whether patients come from particular demographic groups, ask questions, or say they need help to read or understand what physicians tell them, Geri Amori, Ph.D., CPHRM, ARM, director of the Professional Development and Education Center at the Risk Management and Patient Safety Institute, believes it is safe to say that all patients need help to understand their health problems and their choices, including surgical options. And there is no part of the health care experience—from admission history to informed consent to discharge instructions—that does not rely on accurate levels of communication.[3]

It is also in the medical institutions' interests to be sure that all patients understand everything relating to their care. The costs of patients' lack of understanding may include noncompliance with treatment, longer hospital stays, higher health care costs, the opportunity for medical errors, and compromised patient safety.[2]

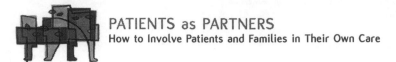

After agreeing to or receiving care, 18% to 45% of patients are unable to recall the major risks of surgery, and many cannot answer basic questions about the services or procedures they agreed to receive.

Effective Written and Verbal Communication

The federal government mandates ensuring patient understanding through clear communication in ways that are tailored to the individual patient. The Centers for Medicare & Medicaid Services (CMS) requires organizations receiving federal funds to comply with civil rights laws prohibiting discrimination against anyone seeking health care services[3,4]:

> ". . . whenever possible, the hospital informs each patient of his or her rights in a language or method of communication that the patient understands. . . . In providing this information, the hospital must be sensitive to the communication needs of its patients. As part of its provider agreement, the hospital agrees . . . that it will provide interpretation for certain individuals who speak languages other than English, use alternative communication techniques or aides for those who are deaf or blind, or take other steps as needed to effectively communicate with the patient. . . . The hospital's obligation to inform requires that the hospital presents information in a manner and form that can be understood, e.g., the use of large print materials, specialized programs to inform individuals who are deaf or blind, use of interpreters, etc. . . . ."

To implement these recommendations, CMS has charged medical institutions to do the following[1]:

- Assess their populations and language needs.
- Develop a written policy for assessing the needs of individual patients with limited English proficiency.
- Provide free language assistance for those with limited English proficiency.
- Identify effective and convenient resources for language assistance and arrange for these services quickly when needed.
- Hire bilingual staff members who are trained and competent in the skill of interpreting (family or friends of the patient should not be used as interpreters).

Tips for Clear Communication

Clear communication is vital in any patient–caregiver relationship but may be particularly challenging when patients have low literacy skills or low health literacy skills. To communicate effectively with patients, it is recommended that physicians take the following steps[1]:

• Communicate with all patients in simple language, without jargon—explain even commonly used medical terms such as *hypertension, terminal,* and *malignant,* because they are not familiar to everyone.[3]

• Limit new concepts to no more than three per visit.

• Use pictures, graphics, real devices, or other visual aids for demonstration.

• Ask questions beginning with "how" and "what" to aid comprehension.

• Slow down and take the time to assess the patient's health literacy skills and understanding.

• Convey information orally and use written material mostly as a backup.[5]

• Go over all written materials with patients, discussing with them the nature and scope of the procedure covered by informed consent forms.

• Provide an interpreter or reader to assist patients with limited English proficiency, visual or hearing impairments, and low literacy skills. ∎

• Translate written materials that are routinely given to patients in English.

• Use informed consent forms written in simple sentences in the primary language of the patient.

Obtaining Informed Consent

Informed consent, and every other aspect of health care, depends on communicating clearly in a language and manner that patients can understand. Clinicians should present information about the proposed treatment, alternative treatments, and the risks and benefits of each—as well as the risks and benefits of no treatment—and discuss these with the patient. Informed consent does not take place when a form is signed; it occurs when patient and physician discuss a problem and choose an intervention together. This process may take place in one sitting or over the course of several appointments. Another term to describe this process is shared decision making.[6,7]

Approaching informed consent discussions, like all medical discussions, requires heightened sensitivity to differences among patients and an understanding of how best to accommodate them. One standard approach will not work for all patients, even under similar clinical circumstances.[7] Clinicians may want to ask patients about their fears, ideas, and expectations at the start of such discussions.[7]

Tip
Clinicians should also be aware of any cultural differences among patients that might guide their interview strategies. For example, "People in many cultures believe that informing the patient of a terminal diagnosis may hasten death. Physicians may be well advised to ask patients, 'How much would you like to know about your illness?' or 'Would you prefer I discuss your diagnosis with your family?'"[8] In some cultures, family members, not patients, are primarily responsible for medical information and decisions, but patients may not make this clear to their physicians. Physicians should ask directly whether this is the case when a major decision needs to be made.[8]

Informed consent discussions can be especially challenging when the patient has low literacy skills or limited English skills. A signed consent form may not be adequate proof of consent if the patient does not have the capacity to understand the information about the risks, benefits, and alternatives to the proposed treatment.[3] The treating physician is responsible not only for informing the patient about the procedure in a language or manner the patient can understand, but also for determining whether the patient has actually understood the information conveyed.[3]

Health care organizations usually develop their own informed consent forms to outline and document the details of the discussions between physicians and patients. These forms tend to use technical or legal language, have several pages of dense text printed in small type, and often don't have space to document that the patient has understood the information discussed.[10] Because most patients are unable to understand or remember the content of the informed consent forms, the National Quality Forum suggests simplifying the forms to the 5th grade reading level or below and using pictures or symbols.[1]

Tip
Patient understanding during informed consent discussions can be enhanced by combining the teach-back method with the use of diagrams. Diagrams seem to be especially important aids in discussions with the elderly.[9]

Physicians' discussions with patients who have low literacy skills or who need special help to understand their medical problems and to make decisions can be difficult, and identifying such patients can be challenging. There are, however, certain populations that will invariably need extra help: children, the elderly, and those with chronic conditions. Communicating with such populations is the subject of Chapter 5.

References

1. Wu H.W., et al.: *Improving Patient Safety Through Informed Consent for Patients with Limited Health Literacy: An Implementation Report.* Washington, DC: National Quality Forum, 2005.

2. Wilson J.F.: The crucial link between literacy and health. *Ann Intern Med* 139:875–878, Nov. 18, 2003.

3. Moore C.: Health care literacy and patient safety: The new paradox. In Youngberg B.J., Hatlie M.J. (eds.): *The Patient Safety Handbook.* Sudbury, MA: Jones and Bartlett, 2004.

4. Center for Medicare & Medicaid Services (CMS): *Appendix A: Regulations and Interpretive Guidelines for Hospitals.* Washington, DC: CMS, Apr. 2004.

5. National Center for the Study of Adult Learning and Literacy: *Insights from Practice and Voices of Experiences.* http://www.hsph.harvard.edu/healthliteracy/insights.html (accessed Dec. 9, 2005).

6. Whitney S.N., McGuire A.L., McCullough L.B.: A typology of shared decision making, informed consent, and simple consent. *Ann Intern Med* 140:54–59, Jan. 6, 2003.

7. Epstein R.M., Alper B.S., Quill T.E.: Communicating evidence for participatory decision-making. *JAMA* 291:2359–2366, May 19, 2004.

8. Personal communication between the writer and Lee Bennett, M.D., Oct. 28, 2005.

9. Misra-Hebert A.D.: Physician cultural competence: Cross-cultural communication improves care. *Cleve Clin J Med* 70:289–303, Apr. 2003.

10. Thompson G.A., et al.: Informed consent: CMS' approach to "minimum expectations." *Health Law Alert* May 2, 2005.

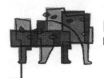

CASE STUDY 4.1
THE IOWA HEALTH SYSTEM HEALTH LITERACY COLLABORATIVE

ARTICLE AT A GLANCE

Name of the organization:
Health Literacy Collaborative, Iowa Health System, Des Moines.

Purpose of the project:
The Iowa Health System sought to develop informed consent forms written at the 7th–8th grade reading level to promote patient understanding, to educate health care providers about the difference between "informed consent" and "consent forms," and to teach providers how to meet Joint Commission and Centers for Medicare & Medicaid Services informed consent requirements.

Lessons learned:
Developing informed consent forms written more simply—at the 7th–8th grade reading level as opposed to the college level—is possible with collaboration by health literacy teams, new readers, adult learners, risk managers, clinicians, and the legal department.

Outcomes:
Although this project is still a work in progress, patients have expressed satisfaction with the new forms, and there has been no increase in the number of patients who have asked for follow-up visits to clarify information.

Staff involved:
Organizational leadership, staff concerned with issues related to health literacy, clinicians, risk managers, and members of the legal department.

A Project to Clarify and Simplify Informed Consent

The Health Literacy Collaborative of the Iowa Health System, under the leadership of Barbara Earles, R.N., M.S., CPHQ, CPHRM, director of Risk Management at the Iowa Health System in Des Moines, has begun to develop informed consent forms written in a language that patients can understand. A driving force behind this project was the collaborative's concerns about issues such as the following:

1. The potential legal ramifications for providers surrounding the issue of health literacy and informed consent—case law addresses the way risk is communicated and recognizes that claims have involved a lack of "informed consent."

2. Consent forms are written in a language that most patients cannot understand—for example, readability analyses from several hospitals in the Iowa Health System revealed that "informed consent" documents were written at the 17th grade level or higher.

3. Consent forms are used as evidence that a conversation took place and informed consent was given.

CASE STUDY 4.1

4. Health literacy is a concern of national attention, involving organizations such as the American Medical Association and the Institute of Medicine.

5. There is a need to meet the standards and regulations of the Joint Commission, the Centers for Medicare & Medicaid Services, the Iowa Code on Informed Consent, the National Quality Forum, and the Leapfrog Group.

What the Iowa Health System Has Done So Far

The Iowa Health System Health Literacy Collaborative has developed a simplified, clear informed consent form to use in place of the standard, difficult-to-read forms that patients are expected to read, understand, and sign before giving their informed consent to surgery. This form was developed in collaboration with all health literacy teams in the Iowa Health System, new readers, adult learners, risk managers, health care providers, surgical services personnel, and the legal department.

The surgical informed consent form was pilot tested and rolled out systematically, one affiliate in the Iowa Health System at a time. Responses were evaluated, data were assessed, and the informed consent process was revised as needed after each step.

In addition to the informed consent form developed for surgical procedures, the Iowa Health System developed another form for procedures involving vaginal birth after caesarian section. Participating in the development of this form were members of health literacy teams, new readers, adult learners, risk managers, obstetrics managers, and the Iowa Health Systems legal department.

Affiliates within the Iowa Health System are now in the process of rewriting and pilot testing informed consent forms that cover anesthesia, conditions of hospital admission, and consent to treatment. All work is done in conjunction with health literacy teams, new readers/adult learners, risk managers, and the legal department.

Three Iowa Health System affiliates have developed the Health Literacy Problem Term Database, now being pilot tested. All medical institutions or clinicians will be able to use this database to identify words that patients may not understand, and to suggest simpler words that will make their informed consent forms easier to understand.

The Iowa Health System plans to translate the final versions of informed consent forms into languages other than English to better serve the needs of a variety of populations.

All work is done in conjunction with health literacy teams, new readers/adult learners, risk managers, and the legal department.

Lessons Learned

Providers, the hospital staff, and—most of all—Iowa Health System patients have expressed significant satisfaction with the simplified surgery/procedure informed consent form. There have been many positive comments about how easy these forms are to read and understand. Patients have not increased their visits back to physicians to clarify procedures since these forms have been in use.

Keys to Success

Key to the success of efforts to simplify informed consent forms is to involve the organization's leadership and everyone who has a role in organizational change.

A second key to success is to educate medical personnel about the difference between "informed consent" and the "consent form." It is the role of the provider to discuss, through a process of shared decision making, the recommended surgery, procedure, treatment plan, anesthesia, or other service. Physicians then need to be sure that patients understand what is being rec-

CASE STUDY 4.1

ommended, the risks and benefits, other options with their risks and benefits, and the risks and benefits of no treatment before their patients make a decision. Providers also should be educated about the need to use simpler language so that all patients will be able to understand what they have agreed to before they sign the form.

A third key to success is to educate the staff involved in risk and quality about the Joint Commission and Centers for Medicare & Medicaid services standards: that all patients must understand, regardless of literacy level or any other consideration, the information contained in consent forms, even if medical institutions need to provide the specific help their patients need. Informed consent is a *process,* not merely a document. Signing of the consent form alone is not sufficient to meet legal requirements for informed consent.

Key Features of the Iowa Health System's Simplified Informed Consent Documents

The following is an example of the way in which the Iowa Health System has transformed difficult-to-understand language in an informed consent form into clear, easy-to-read, and understandable prose:

- **Before:** "It has been explained to me that during the course of the operation, unforeseen conditions maybe revealed that necessitate an extension of the original procedure(s) or different procedure(s) than those described above. I, therefore, authorize such surgical procedure(s) as are necessary and desirable in the exercise of the professional judgment. The authority granted under this shall extend to all conditions that do require treatment even if not known to Dr. _____ at the time the operation is commenced.
- **After:** "I understand the doctor may find other medical conditions he/she did not expect during my surgery or procedure. I agree that my doctor may do any extra treatments or

Informed consent is a process, not merely a document.

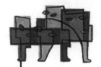
CASE STUDY 4.1

procedures he/she thinks are needed for medical reasons during my surgery or procedure."

The original text was written at the college level; it has been rewritten at 7th–8th grade reading level.

In addition to using simple language, the Iowa Health System simplified the informed consent documents and enhanced their readability by using the following formatting techniques:

- One double-sided page
- 13-point font; Times New Roman
- Layout:
  - Use of white space to avoid text density
  - 1.5–double line-spacing
  - Clear headings
  - Numbering and bullets
  - Purposeful use of bold text
- Lines for recording the procedure in:
  - Medical language AND
  - Patient's own words

More challenges for the Iowa Health System lie ahead. One of the biggest will be to move beyond using a new form to helping providers incorporate "teach-back" methods and to document these discussions in their everyday interactions with patients and families.

PATIENT PERSPECTIVE 4.1
TONI CORDELL,
LITERACY ADVOCATE

Toni Cordell, a literacy advocate from Atlanta, expresses her experiences and her tendencies this way: "The forms are intimidating, yet signing them is mandatory. I sign papers without reading them because I suspect it's mandatory to sign them even if I don't understand them. I let the person at the front desk know I've signed them but I don't understand what I've signed. I think this situation is a lawsuit waiting to happen."

Although her reading skills have improved over the years, she still feels "stupid, intimidated, and resentful" when she goes into a hospital and is confronted with medical forms. Self-conscious of her past poor reading skills and still somewhat defined by them, she never has and still doesn't ask for clarification of the forms: "I have a very hard time asking anyone for anything; I hate asking anyone for help," she says. She believes that, regardless of what the patient is willing or able to ask for, hospitals and clinicians need to provide all patients with the tools they need to understand what they are signing. "If I had a broken leg, you wouldn't ask me to walk up the stairs . . . you would give me a wheelchair," says Cordell.

To help "the hundreds of thousands of people like I was, the one quarter of the population who do not read above the 5th grade level," Cordell says, "I would have liked to have the paperwork sent to me at home a week before surgery. That way, I could at least have looked at the paperwork ahead of time. I could have asked for help from a family member who knows my challenge."

Reading and understanding medical information with the goal of signing forms is only one of Cordell's concerns. Another is the understanding of medical conditions, treatment options, the treatment plan, surgery—in short, all aspects of care whether or

"If I had a broken leg, you wouldn't ask me to walk up the stairs . . . you would give me a wheelchair."

PATIENT PERSPECTIVE 4.1

"He used

his tie

to explain

questions

I had about

changes

in my body

after surgery.

He drew me

pictures.

He took the

time to talk

to me.

I never felt

rushed."

not the signing of forms is involved. So what does she believe is a physician's ideal approach to aid patient understanding? Cordell describes the approach of Neal Galloway, M.D., a urologist at Grady Memorial Hospital in Atlanta, as her ideal communicator: "He sat in a chair facing me and talked to me face-to-face first, while I was still fully clothed. He told me what he was going to do, and what he was doing as he did it. He kept me continually informed. He told me when something would hurt (and he was right). He was kind, considerate, and treated me like a human being both before the exam and after. After the exam, he sat down again in a chair facing me and talked to me face-to-face about what he found. I didn't know what to ask, so he gave me information and then asked me some questions—then I was able to think of questions to ask him. He used his tie to explain questions I had about changes in my body after surgery. He drew me pictures. He took the time to talk to me. I never felt rushed."

Cordell now speaks to medical students at Emory University in Atlanta with the approval of Mark Williams, M.D., who suggests that the students drop the medical vocabulary when they're talking to patients. He says it's fine to talk to colleagues in medical jargon, but one should speak in simple language, in plain English, when talking to patients.

As Cordell emphasizes, "Communication is an opportunity for understanding, or for failure."

CHAPTER FIVE
Addressing the Education
and Involvement Needs
of Special Populations

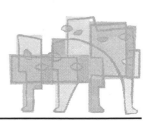

 Every child is different, every parent is

different, every illness or behavior is

somewhat different from any other. . . .

Remember that you know a lot about your

child and that I don't know anything.

Benjamin Spock, M.D.,
BABY AND CHILD CARE

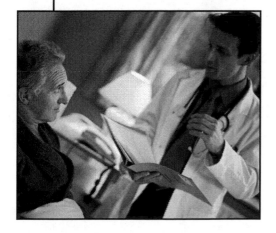

Children, the elderly, and patients with chronic conditions— groups referred to in this chapter as "special populations"— need to participate, like anyone else, as partners in their health care. At the same time, the particular needs of these populations are unique:

• Communicating and partnering with children raises questions about the patient's ability to comprehend and make decisions and poses, at times, complex ethical issues.
• Communicating with elderly patients who may have physical and cognitive impairments requires clinicians to use particular approaches to overcome these obstacles.
• Engaging adults and children who have chronic illnesses not only as partners, but as leaders in managing their health care, requires clinicians to play a supporting role.

The challenges involved in communicating and partnering with patients in these special populations are outlined in this chapter, along with suggested approaches to doing so.

JOINT COMMISSION STANDARDS

PC.6.10 The patient receives education and training specific to the patient's needs and as appropriate to the care, treatment, and services provided.

PC.6.30 The patient receives education and training specific to the patient's abilities as appropriate to the care, treatment, and services provided by the hospital.

The Role of Children and Adolescents in Medical Decision Making

Just as adults differ in their literacy skills, levels of understanding, and need for involvement, children also differ from one another in their capacity to understand and participate in health care decisions. Childhood is a time of continual change, of maturing physically, intellectually, and emotionally. Children mature at different rates, and not all children of the same age will have the ability to make the same types of decisions. Living with a chronic or terminal illness can greatly speed a child's level of maturity. Yet, even when children are capable of making health care decisions, support from their families and clinicians is essential.[1]

Infants and Preschool Children

Infants and children of preschool age are incapable of making significant decisions about their health care. Parents should make decisions on their child's behalf on the basis of what they believe to be in the child's best interests.[1]

Primary School Children

Children of primary school age may participate in medical decisions, although they are incapable of making such decisions on their own, and parents will have to make decisions on their behalf. Clinicians should give children of this age information appropriate to their level of understanding, with an awareness that these children may agree or disagree with a course of action without fully understanding its implications. Clinicians should seek the child's permission for any decisions and should take any strong and prolonged disagreement from the child seriously.[1]

Because young children are unlikely to express or defend their decisions, anxious, stressed, or grieving family members may need the physician's help to focus on what is best for the child. This may be especially difficult when a cure is impossible.[1]

Adolescents

Many adolescents have the same decision-making capacity as adults. As with adults, clinicians should determine an individual adolescent's ability to make health care decisions by assessing his or her ability to do the following[1]:

- Understand and communicate relevant information
- Think and make choices with a degree of independence
- Assess the potential for benefits, risks, and consequences of multiple options

Many children and adolescents, particularly those who have been seriously ill, need help to understand medical issues and show that they are able to make decisions. Teachers, chaplains, play therapists, nurses, psychologists, or others skilled in communicating with children can help.[1]

Involving the Elderly

The National Institute on Aging gives clinicians the following advice for communicating with elderly patients so that this special population of patients is involved as partners involved in its own health care[2]:

On average, clinicians listen to their patients for 18 to 23 seconds before interrupting.

- Establish respect from the outset by using formal terms of address: Mr., Mrs., Ms., and so on.
- Relieve stress by asking friendly questions, such as "Do you have family nearby?" or "Are you active in community programs?"
- Introduce yourself clearly. Show from the start that you accept the patient and want to hear his or her concerns.
- Avoid rushing older patients. Try to give them a few extra minutes to talk about their concerns. As with all patients, doing so will allow you to gather important information and will lead to better cooperation with treatment, saving time in the long run.
- Beware of the patient's tendency to minimize complaints, "not wanting to be a bother," or the patient's concern that he or she is taking up too much of your time.
- Speak slowly to give patients more time to process what is being said.
- Try not to interrupt patients early in the interview. As mentioned in Chapter 2, physicians tend to interrupt patients, on average, within the first 18 to 23 seconds of the initial interview. When interrupted, patients are less likely to reveal all their concerns, which often take more time to clarify.
- Avoid jargon. Use simple, common language and be willing to ask your patients if they understand what you are saying.
- Introduce necessary information by first asking patients what they know about their illness and then building on that.
- Assess vision and hearing problems that can affect communication and need to be treated.

- Speak slowly and clearly in a normal tone.
- Face patients directly, at eye level, and keep your hands away from your face while talking, so they can lip-read or pick up visual clues to what you are saying.
- Tell your patients when you are changing the subject. Give clues such as pausing briefly, speaking a bit more loudly, gesturing toward what will be discussed, gently touching the patient, or asking a question.
- Make sure the setting is adequately lit and that there is enough light on your face.
- Ask whether your patients have brought and/or are wearing the right eyeglasses.
- Make sure your handwritten instructions are easy to read.
- Make sure the type is large enough and the typeface is easy to read when using printed materials.
- Consider using alternatives to printed materials, such as tape-recorded instructions, large pictures or diagrams, or other aids if your patients have trouble reading because of either sensory impairments or low literacy skills.

 Tip Painting, storytelling, writing poetry, or acting may help to open the lines of communication and help clinicians to assess a child's understanding and decision-making ability.[1]

Empowering Patients with Chronic Illness

The health of patients with chronic illness is, like that of other patients, enhanced when they are active participants in their health care, collaborating with clinicians in the process of shared decision making. Communication and problem solving are vital in the partnership between physicians and their patients who are living with chronic illness. The role of clinicians in such partnerships is to empower, support, educate, and help patients with chronic illness in practical ways so they can take the lead in their health care.[4] To achieve these goals, clinicians need to educate themselves about resources currently available to help both themselves and their patients. The Appendix that follows provides practical resources to help clinicians and patients make all the positive changes of which they are capable.

Improving Self-Management Skills

Patients with chronic diseases must take on new self-management skills to improve or maintain their health. These self-management skills require a lifestyle change that can be extremely difficult for patients to accept. Staff members should find out what a particular lifestyle change means to a patient and help the patient want to make the change and see how it can be realized within his or her lifestyle. In addition, staff members must assess their patients' education needs according to their level of acceptance with the lifestyle change. The following tips will help the staff increase a patient's likeliness to adapt to lifestyle changes[5]:

*   Recognize patients as experts in their own lives who are a part of the health care team; doing so can help patients create and agree on short-term action plans (one to two weeks long) that eventually lead to complete lifestyle changes.

Tip Physicians should make an effort to let the patient go on for three to four minutes, and in that time the patient will tell you 90% of what's wrong with him or her.[3]

SIDEBAR 5.1

The Institute for Healthcare Improvement National Program to Advance Patient Self-Management of Care

Patients battling chronic diseases such as asthma, diabetes, hypertension, and HIV have complex and often overlapping medical needs that our health care system has struggled to meet. Pioneering quality experts have developed new tools and strategies to help this population. General and family practice groups increasingly tap into these resources to help their patients with chronic conditions stay healthier, avoid hospitalization, and stay involved with family, work, and community.

Engaging Patients as Partners
"Quality Allies: Improving Care by Engaging Patients," a national program funded by the Robert Wood Johnson Foundation (RWJF) and the California HealthCare Foundation (CHCF), is trying to find ways to involve patients in their care. "We know we need to get more patients more involved in their own care, we just don't know how to do it well," said John Lumpkin, M.D., M.P.H., senior vice president and director of the Health Care Group at RWJF. "By learning how to provide more support for self-management, Quality Allies can help us achieve care for chronic conditions that is more patient-centered."

Self-management support does not come naturally to physicians, according to the Institute for Healthcare

Improvement's Laurel Simmons, deputy director of Quality Allies. "Self-management support is really a new process. It's not about giving patients instructions and lists, telling them what to do for their asthma or congestive heart failure. It's about engaging them as active partners in their treatment." And providers' unease with the process is somewhat understandable, adds Simmons: "Physicians aren't trained to work collaboratively with patients, to communicate and build the right kind of relationship, so they may need new skills and tools."

More information about Quality Allies is available at http://www.ihi.org. ■

- Understand that accomplishment of the action plan is more important than the action plan itself. Patients must start out with realistic goals and then gradually work up to more difficult goals.
- Assess a patient's level of self-efficacy or self-confidence (patients with greater self-efficacy will have improved results). Confidence can be measured by asking specific questions, such as "On a scale of 1 to 10, how confident are you that you can eat one fruit and one vegetable a day and avoid cookies with saturated fats?" If the patient answers with a 7 or higher, it is likely that he or she will succeed; if the patient answers with a 6 or lower, the action plan should be revised so that it is more realistic.
- Assess the patient's management of emotions (that is, their level of uncertainty, fear, depression, loneliness, anger, and stress) and work with the patient on ways to better cope with these emotions or provide them with additional care to address these emotions.

Conclusion

Whether a patient suffers from chronic or acute illness, is an adolescent or an adult, has a graduate school education or an elementary school education, is native to the country in which care is provided or comes from another culture and speaks another language, the research presented in this book resonates with this simple message: It is the role of every clinician and medical institution to ensure patient understanding in every clinical encounter, to encourage and help patients and their families participate actively

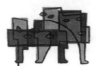
in their care, and to communicate completely, effectively, and clearly with patients and staff alike. Federal and private-sector organizations are conducting much research, as has been described throughout this book, that should provide greater insight into the most effective *ways* to involve patients in their care and what strategies will lead to the best patient outcomes.[6] Results of these studies should be available within the next few years. We fully expect these studies to lead to greater insights about how best to engage patients and families as partners in their care and, in so doing, how to further improve patient safety.

References

1. Harrison C., et al.: Bioethics for clinicians: Involving children in medical decisions. *CMAJ* 156:825–828, Mar. 15, 1997.

2. National Institute on Aging: *Working with Your Older Patient: A Clinician's Handbook.* http://www.niapublications.org/pubs/clinicians2004/index.asp (accessed Dec. 5, 2005).

3. Belzer E.J.: Improving patient communication in no time. *Family Practice Management.* May 1999. http://www.aafp.org/fmp/990500fm/23.html (accessed Sep. 21, 2005).

4. Institute for Healthcare Improvement: *IHI at the Forefront of National Program to Advance Patient Self-Management of Care.* http://www.ihi.org/IHI/Topics/PatientCenteredCare/SelfManagementSupport/ImprovementStories/IHIatForefrontofNationalProgramtoAdvancePatientSelfManagementofCare.htm (accessed Oct. 12, 2005).

5. Bodenheimer T., et al.: Patient self-management of chronic disease in primary care. *JAMA* 288:2469–2475, Nov. 20, 2002.

6. Crawford M.J., et al.: Systematic review of involving patients in the planning and development of health care. *BMJ* 325:1263–1268, Nov. 30, 2002.

PATIENT PERSPECTIVE 5.1

REBECCA BRYSON, MANAGING CHRONIC ILLNESS BY ADVOCATING PATIENT-CENTERED CARE

Rebecca Bryson, of Whatcom County, Washington, is a patient who has had a great deal of experience with the health care system, experiencing chronic illness marked by extensive complications over a period of many years. During the course of her illness and its treatment she has depended on the services of at least 13 health care providers in the fields of family medicine, ophthalmology, gastroenterology, hematology, emergency medicine, cardiology, cardiothoracic surgery, psychology, and pharmacology. Managing her various conditions with so many different providers has been challenging to Bryson, as it is to all patients with chronic illness. Bryson has found that many of the challenges or obstacles facing patients who try to participate in their care stem from the design of a health care system that is "the worst kind of maze, one filled with hazards, barriers, and burdens." For the nearly 100 million Americans who now have one or more chronic illnesses—a number estimated to grow to 134 million by 2020—these systemic failures can have a devastating impact.

Responding to the needs of patients struggling to manage their diseases, especially those with multiple chronic conditions, a group of health care representatives in Whatcom County decided to work together to redesign their care delivery. Participants include the community hospital, a specialty group, clinics, and a physician practice. This collaborative effort was selected to participate in the Robert Wood Johnson Foundation initiative "Pursuing Perfection in Health Care."

Finding ways to help patients better manage their chronic diseases and navigate their way among various health care providers became the focus of Whatcom County's initiative. Early on, it was decided that only by directly involving patients

Patients are

keenly aware

of the lack of

coordination

in care,

and they face

a complex

and often

confusing

delivery

system.

in all redesign efforts could effective solutions be developed. Rebecca Bryson was one of the patients invited to participate.

Bryson, and others participating in the initiative, confirmed two primary concerns: Patients are keenly aware of the lack of coordination in care; and they face a complex and often confusing delivery system.

To address these concerns, health care professionals in Whatcom County developed a new type of health care provider, the clinical care specialist. The Pursuing Perfection grant allowed for the funding of two clinical care specialists in a pilot program. They work directly with patients—each has a case load of about 50—to help coordinate communication and care among a variety of providers and institutions.

To further address problems in communication and coordination, Whatcom County has developed the Shared Care Plan. This single record includes all relevant information about a patient's health, including medications, physicians, and current and previous health conditions. The patient maintains his or her own copy of the Shared Care Plan, and all providers can have access to an electronic version.

Whatcom County's initiatives have been lauded by physicians and patients alike: "Clinical care specialists provide two incredible services. The first one is the most obvious, which is helping a primary care provider and a specialist, or multiple specialists, understand what's happening on either end. They're also able to convert what we say into language the patients can understand so they know what their own responsibilities are," said Dr. Peter Beglin, medical director, Cardiovascular Center, St. Joseph Hospital. As for Bryson: "I've had a number of times where I literally thought I could die today. At those times, without the intervention of Nancy, my clinical care specialist, there's no question in my mind I would not have survived that day."

PATIENT PERSPECTIVE 5.1

This patient-centered program developed in Whatcom County has eased the considerable burden of coordinating care for those who suffer with chronic illnesses. For more information about this program, go to http://www.ramcampaign.org/pages/champ_RBryson.htm.

Source: Crosskeys Media: *It Takes a Community.* http://www.ramcampaign.org/pages/champ_RBryson.htm (accessed Dec. 9, 2005).

PATIENTS as PARTNERS
How to Involve Patients and Families in Their Own Care

APPENDIX
Resources for
Medical Institutions, Clinicians,
and Health Care Consumers

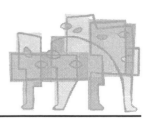

The following organizations' Web sites provide

information for medical institutions, clinicians, and

patients and their families about issues related to patient

safety and patient-centered care. Health care workers can

refer their patients to the information listed in this

Appendix (the specific information for patients and

families is commonly available in English and Spanish).

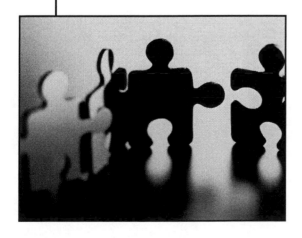

Agency for Healthcare Research and Quality (http://www.ahrq.gov)

The Agency for Healthcare Research and Quality (AHRQ), a branch of the U.S Department of Health and Human Services dedicated to advancing excellence in health care, provides information for professionals and the public on preventing medical errors and promoting patient safety. AHRQ publications are available online or in print, in English and Spanish.

For Patients:

20 Tips to Help Prevent Medical Errors—this fact sheet tells you what you can to do help prevent medical errors. http://www.ahrq.gov/consumer/20tips.htm

20 Tips to Help Prevent Medical Errors in Children—this fact sheet teaches parents how to help their children avoid medical errors. http://www.ahrq.gov/consumer/20tipkid.htm

Check Your Medicines: Tips for Taking Medicines Safely— this checklist can help you avoid medication errors. http://www.ahrq.gov/consumer/checkmeds.htm

Five Steps to Safer Health Care—this fact sheet lists five things you can do to get safer health care. http://www.ahrq.gov/consumer/5steps.htm

Guide to Health Care Quality: How to Know It When You See It— this guide explains how to be a partner in your health care and how to take an active role in making health care decisions. http://www.ahrq.gov/consumer/guidetoq/

Next Steps After Your Diagnosis: Finding Information and Support—this booklet provides support, advice, and information for people who have just been diagnosed with a disease or condition. http://www.ahrq.gov/consumer/diaginfo.htm

Next Steps After Your Diagnosis: The Video—this video helps patients deal with the physical and emotional results of a medical diagnosis. The video informs patients and their families of what they need to know before making treatment decisions and suggests important follow-up questions to ask. http://www.ahrq.gov/consumer/nxtstepvid.htm

Quick Tips—When Getting Medical Tests—this fact sheet helps patients take an active role in making decisions about medical tests and explains how patients should follow up on test results. http://www.ahrq.gov/consumer/quicktips/tiptests.htm

Quick Tips—When Talking with Your Doctor—this fact sheet explains how to give your doctor information, how to get information from your doctor, and what to do when you get home. http://www.ahrq.gov/consumer/5tipseng/5tips.htm

American Academy of Family Physicians (http://www.aafp.org)

The American Academy of Family Physicians (AAFP) provides information for family physicians in a wide range of areas, including clinical care and research, and practice management. AAFP publishes fact sheets for patients and physicians about how to make patients partners in their health care.

For Patients:

Medical Errors: Tips to Help Prevent Them—this fact sheet gives advice on how to prevent medical errors by communicating with your health care team—doctors, nurses, pharmacists—both in and out of the hospital. http://www.familydoctor.org/736.xml

Tips for Talking to Your Doctor—this fact sheet gives tips for talking, asking questions, and following up with your doctor. http://www.familydoctor.org/837.xml

American College of Physicians (http://www.acponline.org)

The American College of Physicians Web site publishes articles of interest to clinicians in the *Annals of Internal Medicine,* online edition.

American Medical Association (http://www.ama-assn.org)

The American Medical Association provides information for clinicians and the general public, with an emphasis on advocacy.

Ask Me Three (http://www.askme3.org)

The Ask Me Three Web site provides three simple, clear tips for talking with your doctor, nurse, or other health care professional.

For Patients:

Tips for Clear Health Communication—this fact sheet tells you what to do when you go to the doctor and how to prepare for the visit. http://www.askme3.org/tips.asp

Chronic Conditions Information Network of Vermont and New Hampshire (http://www.cc-info.net)

This organization helps those who live with or care for those with chronic conditions by providing accurate and relevant health information. The Web site provides links to many resources for patients and their families living with chronic conditions.

For Patients:

Be a Friend with a Pen—this fact sheet gives tips for friends or family members when accompanying someone to the doctor or hospital. http://www.cc-info.net/friend.html

Living with a Chronic Condition—this fact sheet offers support, advice, and links to other resources for people living with chronic illness. http://www.cc-info.net/living.html

Consumers Advancing Patient Safety
(http://www.patientsafety.org)

This organization represents a collective voice for patients, families, and health care professionals wishing to prevent harm in health care encounters through partnership and collaboration.

CRG Medical Foundation
(http://www.communityofcompetence.com)

The CRG Medical Foundation provides information for patients, health care institutions, and clinicians promoting patient safety through communities of competence.

healthfinder® (http://www.healthfinder.gov)

This Web site, sponsored by the U.S. Department of Health and Human Services, provides health care consumers with a gateway to a wide variety of reliable, government-sponsored health information in print and on the Web.

For Patients:

Frequently Asked Questions About Medication Errors—this fact sheet explains what medication errors are and tells how you can help to prevent them. http://www.ismp.org/Pages/ismp_faq.html

Patient Safety Resources—this page links to Web sites and other resources that may be relevant to health care providers and/or patients and families that may have experienced harm due to medical error. http://www.ismp.org/Pages/ismp_faq.html

Institute for Family-Centered Care
(http://www.familycenteredcare.org)

The Institute for Family-Centered Care provides essential leadership to advance the understanding and practice of family-centered care by promoting collaborative, empowering relationships between providers and consumers.

For Patients:

Creating Advisory Councils—this booklet provides practical information about how to set up and run a patient advisory council. http://www.familycenteredcare.org/tools-frame.html

Institute for Healthcare Improvement (http://www.ihi.org)

The Institute for Healthcare Improvement (IHI) works to advance health care quality and delivery. One of the IHI's areas of focus is patient-centered care.

Institute for Safe Medication Practices (http://www.ismp.org)

The Institute for Safe Medication Practices is a health care agency of pharmacists, nurses, and physicians dedicated to learning about medication errors, understanding their system-based causes, and disseminating practical recommendations that can help health care providers, consumers, and the pharmaceutical industry prevent errors.

For Patients:

Consumers' Web page—this Web page includes information on how to take medication safely, how to work as a partner with your doctor, medication history forms, and links to other consumer resources on the Web.
http://www.ismp.org/Pages/Consumer.html

Institute of Medicine (http://www.iom.org)

The Institute of Medicine, through reports such as *To Err Is Human, Crossing the Quality Chasm,* and *Patient Safety: Achieving a New Standard for Care,* poses new challenges for medical institutions and clinicians in the United States.

Joint Commission on Accreditation of Healthcare Organizations (http://www.jcaho.org)

The Joint Commission on Accreditation of Healthcare Organizations is a private, not-for-profit organization dedicated to continuously improving the safety and quality of care provided to the public. The Joint Commission is the nation's principal standards setter and evaluator for a variety of health care organizations, including hospitals, critical access hospitals, ambulatory care organizations, behavioral health care organizations, home care organizations, laboratories, and long term care organizations.

For Patients:

Speak Up Initiatives—In March 2002 the Joint Commission launched a new patient safety campaign called Speak Up. The aim of these campaigns is to encourage patients to become an informed and active member of the health care team. Brochures have been created on the following topics to improve and urge patient involvement in the health care process:

Speak Up: Help Prevent Errors in Your Care—this brochure provides simple advice on how you, as the patient, can make your care a positive experience. http://www.jcaho.org/general+public/gp+speak+up/speakup_poster.pdf

Help Prevent Errors in Your Care: For Surgical Patients—this brochure offers tips that can help you prepare for surgery and make sure that you have the correct procedure performed at the correct place, or site, on your body. http://www.jcaho.org/general+public/gp+speak+up/wrong_site_brochure.pdf

Preparing to Be a Living Organ Donor—this brochure provides information that can help you, as a potential living organ donor, prepare for surgery and the best possible recovery. http://www.jcaho.org/general+public/gp+speak+up/donor_brochure.pdf

Three Things You Can Do to Prevent Infection—this brochure provides information on three easy things you can do to fight the spread of infection and thus avoid contagious diseases like the common cold, strep throat, and influenza. http://www.jcaho.org/general+public/gp+speak+up/infection_control_brochure.pdf

Things You Can Do to Prevent Medication Mistakes—this brochure provides basic information to help prevent a medication mistake from happening to you or your loved ones. http://www.jcaho.org/general+public/gp+speak+up/speakup_brochure_meds.pdf

Planning Your Recovery—this brochure provides guidance that will ensure you have all the discharge information that is necessary to your quick recovery. http://www.jcaho.org/general+public/gp+speak+up/speakup_recovery.pdf

What You Should Know About Research Studies—this brochure provides guidance and a list of questions to ask if you're thinking about participating in a clinical research study. http://www.jcaho.org/general+public/gp+speak+up/speakup_research.pdf

The Kenneth B. Schwartz Center Rounds (http://www.theschwartzcenter.org/rounds.asp)

This program for health professionals is designed to enhance and support improved communications and strengthen relationships between clinicians and patients and among clinicians themselves.

Massachusetts Coalition for the Prevention of Medical Errors (http://www.macoalition.org)

The coalition increases awareness of error prevention strategies through public and professional education, focusing on initiatives that can best improve patient care.

For Patients:
Your Role in Safe Medication Use: A Guide for Patients and Families—this booklet gives guidance to patients and family members about how to ensure safe medication use.
http://www.macoalition.org/documents/ConsumerGuide.pdf

Medically Induced Trauma Support Services, Inc. (MITSS) (http://www.mitss.org)

MITSS supports, educates, trains, and offers assistance to individuals affected by medically induced trauma.

National Council on Patient Information and Education (NCPIE) (http://www.talkaboutrx.org/index.jsp)

One of the original patient safety coalitions, NCPIE works to advance the safe, appropriate use of medicines through enhanced communication.

For Patients:
Prescription Pain Medicines: What You Need to Know—this full-color brochure features practical advice to support safe use of prescription pain medicines. It includes recognition and management of side effects, patient responsibilities, and tips on using opioid pain medicines wisely. http://www.talkaboutrx.org/educational_resources.jsp?catalog_num=%23B-18

National Family Caregivers Association (http://www.nfcacares.org)

The National Family Caregivers Association supports, empowers, educates, and speaks up for the more than 50 million Americans who care for a chronically ill, aged, or disabled loved one.

For Patients:
Tips and Guides—these tip sheets and how-to guides help family caregivers deal with the emotional and practical sides

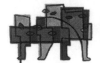

of caregiving. Included are links to fact sheets that help patients and caregivers communicate effectively with health care professionals. http://www.thefamilycaregiver.org/ed

National Institute on Aging (http://www.niapublications.org)

The National Institute on Aging, a branch of the National Institutes of Health, U.S. Department of Health and Human Services, supports research and disseminates information on aging and health for physicians and health care consumers.

For Patients:

Choosing a Doctor—this fact sheet explains what older people should look for in a doctor, and how to choose the right one. http://www.niapublications.org/engagepages/choose.asp

Hospital Hints—this fact sheet explains what to expect when a hospital stay is needed. It explains how to plan, what members of the health care team do, patient rights, and more. http://www.niapublications.org/engagepages/hospital.asp

Medicines: Use Them Safely—this fact sheet includes information about what to tell and ask your doctor, what to ask your pharmacist, and what you need to do to ensure that you take medicines safely. http://www.niapublications.org/engagepages/medicine.asp

Online Health Information: Can You Trust It?—this fact sheet explains how to find reputable, respected sources of health information on the Web. http://www.niapublications.org/engagepages/healthinfo.asp

National Patient Safety Foundation (http://www.npsf.org)

The National Patient Safety Foundation raises public awareness and fosters communication about patient safety.

For Patients:

What You Can Do to Make Health Care Safer—fact sheets about the following:

- What you can do to prevent infections in the hospital
- The role of the patient advocate
- Safety as you go from hospital to home
  http://www.npsf.org/html/publications.html#bro

National Quality Forum (http://www.nqf.org)

The National Quality Forum is an organization dedicated to developing and implementing a national strategy for health care quality measurement and reporting.

Partnership for Patient Safety (P4PS) (http://www.p4ps.org)

P4PS is a patient-centered initiative that initiates focused partnerships and joint ventures with organizations and individuals to achieve a health care system that is patient-centered and systems-based.

Persons United in Limiting Standards and Errors (PULSE) (http://www.pulseamerica.org)

PULSE is dedicated to raising awareness about patient safety and reducing medical errors through advocacy, education, and support.

Risk Management Foundation (RMF) (http://www.rmf.harvard.edu)

RMF is an internationally renowned leader in evidence-based risk management. RMF supports physicians, office practices, and patient safety services; provides litigation management and defense of malpractice claims; and uses claims-based research and data to provide decision support for health care leaders.

Sorry Works! Coalition (http://www.sorryworks.net)

The Sorry Works! Coalition is an organization of doctors, insurers, lawyers, hospital administrators, patients, and researchers joining together to provide a "middle ground" solution to the medical malpractice crisis.

Voice for Patients (http://www.voice4patients.com)

Voice for Patients is an organization for patients, families, and the general public offering informative online resources, including a list of disease-specific organizations that offer support and education, and resources for the victims of medical error, surviving family members, and patient advocates.

For Patients:

Patient Literature—this section links to a variety of resources and publications for the general public.
http://www.voice4patients.com/patient_literature.htm

Whatcom County Pursuing Perfection Project (http://www.ramcampaign.org)

The goal of *Remaking American Medicine* is to inspire and empower the public by demonstrating what transforming the quality of patient care can mean to all Americans.

For Patients:

Remaking American Medicine: Improving the Quality of Health Care Community by Community—this brief report explains how all citizens can get involved in improving health care quality and making patient-centered care the standard of care. The report includes links to many organizations and online resources. http://www.ramcampaign/org/pages/RAM.org_White_Paper.htm

INDEX

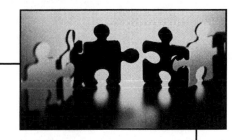